ABOUT THE AUTHOR

Dr Katy Munro worked as a GP in the NHS for over 30 years. During this time, she became a person with migraine, which made her passionate about helping others with this condition. She became a headache specialist GP at the National Migraine Centre, a charity providing people with migraine access to high-quality care. She is also a member of the Council of the British Association for the Study of Headaches.

Dr Munro was instrumental in starting the *Heads Up* podcast which she co-hosts to educate and give advice to anyone with, or caring for, a person with migraine. She is also a spokesperson on migraine, having been interviewed on the BBC, ITV and by numerous journalists. She has been a guest on podcasts including the *Liz Earle Wellbeing Show* and *The Doctor's Kitchen* podcast.

PENGUIN LIFE EXPERTS SERIES

The Penguin Life Experts series equips readers with simple but vital information on common health issues and empowers readers to get to know their own bodies to better improve their health. Books in the series include:

Managing Your Migraine
by Dr Katy Munro

* * * * *

Preparing for the Perimenopause and Menopause
by Dr Louise Newson

* * * * *

Next in the series, publishing in 2021 and 2022:

Keeping Your Heart Healthy
by Dr Boon Lim

* * * * *

Understanding Allergy
by Dr Sophie Farooque

* * * * *

Managing IBS
by Dr Lisa Das

Managing Your Migraine

DR KATY MUNRO

PENGUIN LIFE

AN IMPRINT OF

PENGUIN BOOKS

PENGUIN LIFE

UK | USA | Canada | Ireland | Australia
India | New Zealand | South Africa

Penguin Life is part of the Penguin Random House group of companies
whose addresses can be found at global.penguinrandomhouse.com.

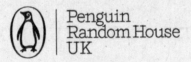

First published 2021

002

Copyright © Dr Katy Munro, 2021

The moral right of the author has been asserted

Set in 11.8/14.75 pt Garamond MT Std
Typeset by Jouve (UK), Milton Keynes
Printed and bound in Great Britain by Clays Ltd, Elcograf S.p.A.

The authorized representative in the EEA is Penguin Random House Ireland,
Morrison Chambers, 32 Nassau Street, Dublin D02 YH68

A CIP catalogue record for this book is available from the British Library

ISBN: 978-0-241-51428-3

www.greenpenguin.co.uk

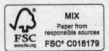

MIX
Paper from
responsible sources
FSC   www.fsc.org   FSC® C018179

Penguin Random House is committed to a
sustainable future for our business, our readers
and our planet. This book is made from Forest
Stewardship Council® certified paper.

Contents

To migraine warriors
and their support teams everywhere

Introduction

Migraine is one of the most common, most prevalent and most debilitating conditions in the world, yet it is widely misunderstood, stigmatized and far too often dismissed as 'just a headache'. Migraine is much more than a headache. It is a genetic, neurological brain disorder affecting people in a variety of ways.

One in seven people suffers from migraine. Three times as many women have migraine attacks as men, and 8 per cent of children have them too. Migraine accounts for 89 per cent of headaches experienced worldwide.[1] Unfortunately, however, many adults and children never receive a formal diagnosis and, without this, miss out on treatment options for managing their symptoms. Many lose days every year, or every month, to this condition.

The World Health Organization's Global Burden of Diseases, Injuries and Risk Factors (GBD) study measures disease impact and helps governments and organizations identify and plan health-service priorities. The GBD ranks migraine as the second-highest cause of disability in the world, right after lower back pain. As recently as 2016, GBD researchers said that 'effective strategies to modify the course of headaches and alleviate pain exist, but many people affected by headache are not benefiting from this knowledge'.[2]

And migraine attacks do not just affect the individual. Their impact spreads out in ripples to family, friends and colleagues and has a huge economic impact on our society. A 2018 report by the Work Foundation revealed that 86 million workdays are lost every year in the UK due to migraine-related absenteeism (sick leave) and presenteeism (reduced effectiveness at work). Migraine costs the UK economy up to £9.7 billion a year.[3] In the US the annual cost of healthcare and absenteeism is $8,294 higher for people with migraine, and headache is the fourth most common reason that people go to hospital emergency departments.[4] And when migraine becomes chronic, the economic burden increases: medical costs in the EU for people with chronic migraine have been found to be three times higher than for those with episodic migraine.[5]

Many doctors lack training in migraine diagnosis and treatment. There's also a lack of research funding. To help people with migraine live their lives more fully it is crucial to improve the understanding of migraine and the strategies available to manage it.

Looking for answers

With one in seven people suffering from migraine attacks, it's likely that you're either a person with migraine or know one. You may have come to this book hoping to find explanations, solutions, maybe even a cure. Because migraine is a genetic, neurological brain disorder, a cure is not a realistic goal. But with the right information and support, the impact of migraine can be greatly relieved.

I first became passionate about spreading good-quality information about migraine and better ways to manage attacks about twenty years ago. I was working as a GP in a busy practice in London when I realized the headaches I was having every week were in fact migraine. I was in my early forties and had not previously had troublesome headaches. Having missed lunch after a packed morning surgery had spilled over into the afternoon, my head seemed to pound and throb as I walked slowly downstairs. I remember standing there, gazing at piles of letters to read, prescriptions to sign and home-visit lists to review and wondering how I'd ever manage the rest of the day. The pain was blinding; it was hard work to think. Once I recognized that my diagnosis was migraine, I was able to take the first steps to finding an effective treatment plan.

As part of my search, I visited the National Migraine Centre, a charity offering appointments with headache-specialist doctors. Inspired by my experience of coming to understand and manage my own migraine, I later joined the team of doctors working at the centre. In addition to seeing patients, I also helped create and present our *Heads Up* podcast, with the goal of getting clear information to more people with migraine.

In this book I'll share the explanations, solutions and treatments we currently have for migraine. I'll explain what migraine is, what can trigger an attack and what can be done to help treat or prevent it. I'll look at some of the newer, safer and better-tolerated treatments that are now becoming available too. Some patients receiving these exciting new treatments describe them as life-changing.

Talking about migraine

First, let's understand some common terms.

Doctors classify headache conditions under two main

headings: primary headaches and secondary headaches.[6] **Primary headaches** are those that are a disorder in themselves. They are not caused by something else. **Secondary headaches** are those with an underlying cause: for example, an infection like meningitis, a tumour or bleeding in the brain. Migraine is classified as a primary headache disorder, even if you don't experience it as head pain.

Migraine is divided into two subtypes based on the frequency of your attacks:

- **Episodic migraine** comes in attacks that resolve completely for some time.
- **Chronic migraine** comes in attacks that occur on more than fifteen days a month.

It is also divided into two other subtypes,[7] based on the effects you feel:

- **Migraine with aura** involves symptoms starting and settling within the hour before the main attack. These are often, but not exclusively, visual changes. People describe seeing zigzag lines, sparkles or shimmers. Some even lose vision completely. Only about 25 per cent of people with migraine get aura.
- **Migraine without aura** enters the headache phase without these aura effects. About 75 per cent of people with migraine don't get aura.

Sometimes people get both types. They may have one type earlier in life and another later on, or they may fluctuate between the two.

The words we use when talking about migraine are

important. The stigma of migraine goes back centuries. From the Victorian era into the twentieth century it was considered to be a nervous condition associated with weakness and neurotic tendencies.[8] Now that we know more clearly what causes migraine, we should choose our words carefully to avoid sustaining outdated stigmas.

I prefer to talk about 'people with migraine' in this book, rather than using terms like 'migraineur' or 'migraine sufferer', to avoid defining people by their diagnosis. Talking about 'migraines' can diminish the recognition of migraine as a neurological condition, so I talk about 'migraine attacks'. People sometimes tell me they have 'cluster migraine'. This misleading term confuses two distinct medical conditions: chronic migraine, where attacks occur frequently, and cluster headache, a separate disorder requiring different treatment.

Listening to family histories in my migraine clinic, I sometimes hear patients say, 'She had just the normal headaches everyone gets.' This is not, in fact, true. Not everyone gets headaches, and if they do have them, then a proper diagnosis is incredibly useful in finding the right treatments. Plus, migraine attacks can vary in severity and don't always cause severe headache pain. Some bring intense dizziness; others cause weakness of one side of the body. Misconceptions around this neurological condition are very common. By clarifying these, we can work to a better understanding of what is happening to us and how we can manage it well.

So let's start your mission to understand migraine.

1. Are You a Person with Migraine?

If you're reading this book, you or someone you care about is probably experiencing symptoms that you think might be migraine. You may be wondering: What should I look out for? When should I see a doctor? How will my doctor know whether my symptoms are migraine? Should I be having tests?

As many as 25 per cent of people with migraine never get a diagnosis, even when they visit a doctor.[1] There are many others who never even go and ask. This needs to change. The first step is to understand what migraine is and how you personally experience it. You need to prepare and tell the story of your symptoms.

What symptoms do you get?

Migraine is classically thought of as a one-sided severe headache with vomiting and sensitivity to light. While often true, this is certainly not the whole story. Migraine symptoms vary in number, type, frequency, duration and severity. Your symptoms can change from attack to attack or across the course of your life.

Let's consider some of the symptoms people with migraine can experience.

- **Headache**: This is often described as throbbing, pounding or pulsating. It typically worsens with movement, giving a banging sensation. Pain can be felt anywhere on the head – either side, at the front, at the back or all over. It may move around during an attack. It may be felt in the jaw or sinuses. Not all migraine attacks result in headache, however.

- **Neck or shoulder pain**: Neck and shoulder pains are common and can be felt on their own or at the start of a migraine attack, with pain then travelling up over the back of the head. Pain travelling in the opposite direction, from the head down to the neck and shoulders, can also happen.

- **Visual disturbances**: These might be flashing or sparkling lights, blurred vision or zigzag patterns in black-and-white or colour. Others notice blind spots in the centre of their vision (scotomata). Disturbances usually occur in both eyes but, rarely, with retinal migraine (see Chapter 12) may be on one side only. When they come and go within an hour before the main attack they are typical of migraine aura.

- **Sensory sensitivities**: The brain of a person with migraine cannot properly process sensory inputs from external stimulation, such as light, sound, smells or touch, even when an attack isn't happening. For example, you may hate TVs on in different rooms with sounds clashing, or can't tolerate sunlight flickering through leaves on a car journey.

- **Skin sensitivity (allodynia)**: This is heightened sensitivity of the skin, especially the scalp. For example, you may find gently brushing your hair or even just touching your skin feels sore. It happens more in people with frequent migraine attacks and chronic migraine.

- **Nausea or vomiting**: This varies from mild to severe and sudden, but is not always present. When it occurs, it may cause problems in keeping down painkillers.
- **Abdominal pain**: This tends to come in attacks with a clear start and stop and is usually felt around the belly button or all round the abdomen. The pain can last between one and seventy-two hours. Sometimes it's so severe it prevents normal daily activities. It may or may not be linked with headache at the same time. Abdominal pain seems to occur in 4–9 per cent of children.[2] It is less common in adults.
- **Gut effects**: Sometimes there is also diarrhoea or bloating.
- **Pale skin (pallor)**: People with headache or abdominal pain can look noticeably pale, with dark rings below their eyes during or after attacks.
- **'Brain fog'**: Those with migraine often describe difficulty in thinking clearly during an attack. Migraine affects their concentration, problem-solving skills, memory or speed of thinking.
- **Speech difficulties**: Sometimes people in an acute attack struggle to speak clearly, experiencing slurred speech or problems finding words.
- **Numbness or tingling of the face or limbs**: This usually occurs on one side of the body. It may involve just one or two areas or run all down one side.
- **Dizziness**: This may be an occasional symptom or a severe, disabling loss of balance, as in vestibular migraine (see Chapter 12).
- **Disturbed sleep**: Pain from migraine may wake people through the night.

- **Yawning and fatigue**: These commonly occur before, during or after the headache. People describe feeling drained or utterly exhausted.
- **Slowing down of functioning**: People with migraine have described this to me as 'walking through treacle' and 'my limbs feel leaden'. Often this slowing down is hard to put into words. Many people struggle to describe it.
- **Mood changes**: Irritability, anxiety and low mood can all occur as part of an attack. Some people feel very depressed during an attack but their mood returns to normal soon after the attack has resolved. When migraine becomes chronic, however, it is common for the impact on daily living to bring anxiety and even clinical depression. There's a lot of help available, so if your mental well-being is suffering because of migraine, please talk to your doctor.

It's really not 'just a headache'

This long list of symptoms is why many people with migraine get so annoyed when their condition is dismissed as 'just a headache'. Migraine headaches range in severity and may not even be the most difficult symptom a person is having.

Which is your most bothersome symptom? Does it change?

Becoming more aware of your symptoms will help you tell the story of your migraine to your doctor or headache specialist. Assumptions that it's 'all about the headache' may lead you down a treatment pathway that isn't right for you.

There is also a commonly held belief that 'true migraine' must result in the person taking to their bed and being completely unable to function. This is simply not true. Many people with migraine try hard to push through their pain and carry on with daily activities – occasionally with the help of painkillers, often by sheer determination! This is why some people with migraine refer to themselves as 'migraine warriors'.

Sadly, because symptoms of migraine are invisible and impossible to test for, people with migraine have often been dismissed, disbelieved or stigmatized. Some people with migraine mistakenly think their symptoms don't merit medical attention. I'm here to tell you they do.

Keeping a migraine diary

A **migraine diary** will help you tell the story of your attacks when you meet your doctor or headache specialist. Your history is key to making a diagnosis, since there are no tests for migraine. How your symptoms started originally, what other effects and sensitivities you get, any patterns in your attacks, how work affects your migraine, any triggers you might have noticed and what helps (and doesn't help) are all clues to aid you and your doctor or headache specialist monitor and treat your condition. In the Further Reading and Resources (see page 211) you can find downloadable migraine diaries and apps, which many of my patients at the National Migraine Centre have found useful. Alternatively, you can make your own month-by-month chart or spreadsheet.

No matter what diary you use, keep it simple:

- **Date, day of the week and time**: Record the days on which you have an attack each month and about what time of day each attack started.

- **Pain**: Rank the severity of any pain or other symptoms in a way that has meaning for you. Some people find a 1–10 scale works (where 10 is the most severe), while others prefer using three categories like 'mild/moderate/severe' or 'green/amber/red'.
- **Medications**: Note what medications you took (if any) and what time of day you took them. A simple code can be quicker – for example, A for aspirin or I for ibuprofen.
- **Big events**: Mark relevant events that might be making your migraine worse – stressful occurrences, travel, parties, menstrual cycle, etc.

You don't need to specify what you ate at each meal – the simpler and quicker your diary is to fill in, the more likely you are to keep it up. Remember to take it with you to appointments.

Who gets migraine?

Migraine attacks can occur throughout childhood, adulthood and even into old age. Boys and girls have the same incidence until puberty, but migraine is three times more common in girls and women as they move into adulthood. In women it tends to be more common in the reproductive years, between puberty and the menopause.[3] After the menopause, attacks usually become less troublesome.

The condition is seen around the world, with one billion people each year experiencing at least one migraine attack.[4] While researchers have not identified any strong ethnic predispositions to migraine, local conditions – such as bright, glaring sunlight or poor air quality from pollution – can have an effect. Migraine attacks may be more common in people with lower income or a poorer education, but it is not clear if these make people more susceptible to migraine or result from migraine disrupting school or work.

One thing is clear: migraine is a genetic disorder that runs in families.

Many genes contribute to migraine and can be passed down the generations. So far, researchers have identified at least thirty-eight different places on chromosomes of genes probably associated with migraine.[5] The influence of genes is higher for certain types of migraine, including migraine with aura.

Researchers believe that genetic influences cause alterations to the brain's sensitivity, making it more prone to irritation by sensory inputs, including noise, light, smell and touch. The migraine brain is more sensitive to other changes too. Changing stress or hormone levels, falling blood glucose, poor sleep patterns, stuffy air quality, weather changes and other factors can all affect the brain of a person with migraine.

Your environment also plays a part by switching certain inherited genes on or off, a process called **epigenetics**. This affects your chances of actually developing migraine attacks if you have inherited the genes. The 'expression' of genes – meaning how cells use information in genes to guide their response to incoming signals – varies from person to person and throughout life. This is why migraine is said to be a **fluctuating condition**, where susceptibility to attacks can wax and wane; and a **spectrum condition**, where severity varies widely.

Your family history

Knowing whether people in your family also have, or had, a history of migraine can be a valuable clue for you and your doctor. Think about your siblings, parents, grandparents, aunts and uncles. Which of them may have had migraine symptoms? Migraine is more common in women, and I often hear women recalling that their mother had it, and their mother's mother before her too.

If you seem to be the only person in your family to have migraine, that doesn't mean you don't have a family history, however. There are several reasons why you may not know of a family history of migraine.

In the past, many people with recurrent severe headaches and vomiting were labelled as suffering from 'sick' or 'bilious' headaches. Sometimes migraine headaches were misdiagnosed as tension headache or sinusitis, or not diagnosed at all. People who were adopted may have no knowledge of their birth parents' medical history. Perhaps your relatives, like some of my patients, have simply never asked, or been asked about their attacks.

When I'm talking to adult patients with migraine about family history, I remind them to think about their children too. With a strong family history of migraine – for example, a parent or sibling with migraine – there is a tendency for migraine to start at a younger age. Unfortunately, children and grandchildren may get migraine more severely, with more frequent attacks. They also seem to have an increased likelihood of having migraine with aura.

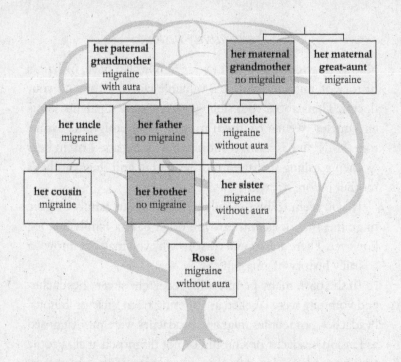

How you may have inherited your migraine

If one parent suffers from migraine, there is a 50 per cent chance of their child having it. If both parents have migraine, the chance increases to 75 per cent.

Rose's story

Rose is twenty-six. She gets migraine without aura, especially if she's very busy, sleeping badly and skipping meals due to pressure of work and then has some alcohol. Her sister, aged thirty-two, also has migraine without aura. This started at university. She noticed it went away during her pregnancy. Their brother and father have never had migraine attacks.

Rose's mother started getting headaches at work in her late forties, when she was often working long hours and missing meals. She blamed the onset of the menopause. Rose's grandmother on her mother's side did not have migraine, but her sister, Rose's great-aunt, had migraine very severely.

On Rose's father's side, her grandmother had headaches – 'one of my heavy heads' as she described them – throughout her life, and still occasionally, but mildly, at the age of ninety. When she was younger, she'd notice visual changes about an hour before her headache – migraine with aura. One of Rose's father's brothers has migraine, and so does his daughter.

Chat with relatives to uncover your own family history and genetic legacy.

When to speak to your doctor

You may have once managed mild headache symptoms with simple painkillers that you bought at the shops without a prescription. Maybe, as things got worse, you had an eye check to see if eye strain was the problem. But there comes a time when you need to seek advice from a doctor.

If you're experiencing sudden severe headache, weight loss,

high fever, collapsing, confusion or weakness, you need a full investigation to establish the cause. Get urgent medical advice if you have any of these symptoms, or trouble speaking or seeing. Don't put up with symptoms that are unexplained.

Arrange a consultation with your doctor if:

- Your headaches are increasing in frequency or severity, or lasting longer
- Simple treatments just don't work
- Your symptoms interrupt your sleep, daily activities or work
- You have other bothersome symptoms, such as nausea, vomiting or dizziness
- You have noticed that light, sound or movement makes things worse.

Your migraine diary and notes will help you tell the story of your attacks when you meet your doctor or headache specialist. Be sure to take them with you to your appointments. Too many of the headache diaries that my patients fill out get left on the kitchen table!

'Surely I need a brain scan?'

People sometimes arrive in my migraine clinic feeling frustrated. They have been having migraine attacks for some time and have struggled to find a helpful treatment. They have spoken to their GP and expected that tests would find out what's wrong, but they haven't been referred for them. Or they've had a brain scan or blood tests and the results haven't helped. Are more tests needed? The short answer is: there are no tests that can identify migraine.

What tests *can* establish is whether something else might be causing your symptoms.

Often the doctor who first sees a person with headache will check their blood pressure and do a neurological examination. During this, the functioning of the cranial nerves in your head, as well as your reflexes, gait, balance, strength and sensation in your limbs, is checked. They'll look at the back of your eyes (the fundus) with an ophthalmoscope, to see if your optic nerves look normal.

Some blood tests can be useful to exclude other causes of headache, such as giant cell arteritis (GCA) (see Chapter 13). However, no blood tests can prove that someone has migraine.

If a doctor believes a brain scan might be useful for excluding other conditions, you'll typically have either a CT or an MRI scan.

CT scans use specialist X-ray equipment to take images from different angles and combine them into a detailed cross-sectional picture showing the blood vessels, bones and soft tissues. These can show if bleeding has occurred in the brain, or if there are signs of stroke, a tumour or skull deformities. **CT angiography** is a more specialized scan, looking for bulges in blood vessels in the brain (aneurysms) that might rupture and cause bleeding.

MRI scans use strong magnetic pulses and radiofrequency waves to create a detailed cross-sectional picture of the area scanned. MRI scans can be useful to look for tumours, aneurysms and some neurological conditions. These show the structure of the brain but can't tell us how it's working, so migraine does not show up. The issue with the brain in a person with migraine has more to do with function – how the brain is responding to a perceived overload of sensory inputs. Comparing the brain to a computer, you could say that the problem isn't the 'hardware' but rather the 'software'.

Brain scans carry risks too. Some people experience claustrophobia in an MRI scanner; having X-rays too often can increase cancer risk later in life; and about one in four scans picks up abnormalities that are 'red herrings' – nothing to do with the person's symptoms (which is why they are sometimes nicknamed 'incidental-omas'). The fact that something showed up raises unnecessary anxiety in both patient and doctor, especially where the abnormality doesn't require treatment.

Could it be something else?

You and your doctor may quickly be sure that your attacks are due to migraine, but sometimes the diagnosis may not be so obvious. There are some important conditions that can cause headaches or be mistaken for migraine. If your symptoms and family history aren't in line with a migraine diagnosis, then you and your doctor may want to consider other possibilities. Chapter 13 goes into more detail about some of these.

Many of my patients have told me that they have seen a variety of other doctors before meeting me. They have been treated with antibiotics for suspected sinusitis, had dental work, been sent for investigations of dizziness or rushed to an emergency department for a lumbar puncture or scan, to rule out infection or a bleed in the brain. Some have been treated for years for migraine but in fact they have cluster headache – an excruciatingly painful condition that is distinct from migraine, though it has some similarities.

The different causes of headache can, however, be clarified through careful history-taking. This is another reason why it helps so much if you're able to describe all your symptoms, and how they have affected you, when you go to see your doctor.

Red flags!

There are times when a brain scan is completely appropriate, and even urgent, to exclude other conditions. Doctors call these 'red flags'. Here are some important ones:

- A very severe, sudden-onset headache that feels like a 'thunderclap' – this requires urgent medical attention at an emergency department.
- A new headache – especially in a child, during pregnancy, at age fifty-five or older or after a recent injury.
- A change in headache – particularly if the person is pregnant or has previously had cancer, or has problems with blood clotting.
- Worrying aspects of a headache – for example, if onset comes with a change of posture, or if there is a possibility of an infection like meningitis or HIV.

All new and changing headaches need to be taken seriously, with an assessment done by a suitably experienced healthcare professional in a GP's surgery or hospital.

Learning about your diagnosis

If you're having symptoms that line up with a migraine attack, the chances are you have migraine. Welcome to the club: there are many of us with it. But don't worry – learning more about your migraine will help you manage your attacks, and I'm happy to say that we have a lot more information about migraine today than we did a generation ago.

Discoveries about the genes and pain chemicals associated with migraine have led to a better understanding of what's happening in the brain during each phase of an attack, including the role of sensory inputs as triggers. In the next chapter we'll look at the condition of migraine in more detail to help you minimize its impact on your life.

2. Understanding Phases and Triggers

'If only I knew what triggers my migraine attacks!' is a recurrent and plaintive cry I hear in my clinics. It's one thing knowing that your brain is more easily irritated by sensory inputs, and another to manage life in a world full of them. The search for triggers can be frustrating, particularly because many people are looking for things at the wrong time – shortly before or when the headache starts. Your attack probably started well before then.

That's because a migraine attack has four phases. Although a brain scan can't prove a diagnosis of migraine, researchers have been able to observe changes in brain activity in people having a migraine attack using **functional MRI scanners**, which detect changes in the flow of blood to different areas of the brain as nerve cells (neurons) activate.[1]

Functional MRI scans show that neurons in two particular areas are active during a migraine attack. One of these areas is the hypothalamus, a small area at the base of the brain involved in releasing hormones and regulating several automatic body processes like body temperature, heart rate, appetite and waking and sleeping patterns. The other area is the brainstem, which connects the brain to the spinal cord and the main nerves of the face and neck – nerves that sense vision, sounds, smells and tastes. The brainstem is also crucial in controlling automatic body processes. Scans have shown that these areas start to present a pattern like the one seen during a migraine well before the headache starts, and these changes may persist for some time after the headache has gone.

The four phases of migraine can blur together if your attacks become more frequent, with one rolling into another. Still, it's useful to consider each phase, one by one, since they build up, getting larger, like a handful of snow rolling across more snow, growing into a bigger and bigger snowball. Migraine attacks can snowball when you don't treat them early, or if the treatments you try aren't effective.

Phase 1 – premonition

A migraine attack can start any time between two and seventy-two hours before you're fully aware of it. When asked to think back on their attacks, about 77–87 per cent of people recall symptoms in this first phase,[2] technically called the **prodrome** or **premonitory phase**. People with migraine with aura and hemiplegic migraine (see Chapter 12) are more likely to report symptoms in this phase. The worse your attack, the more likely you are to have some symptoms in this phase.

Premonitory symptoms tend to develop gradually. I think of this phase as a small snowball beginning to roll down a hill, snow sticking to it as it travels.

> **Symptoms you might notice in the premonitory phase**
> The first seven symptoms below are those most commonly reported:
>
> • **Fatigue, weariness and drowsiness**

- Neck stiffness
- Increased sensitivity to light (photophobia) or sounds (phonophobia)
- Blurred vision
- Yawning
- Skin looking pale (pallor)
- Cravings for certain foods
- Stomach ache (abdominal discomfort)
- Passing urine in large volumes (polyuria)
- Dizziness, vertigo or light-headedness
- Loss of appetite
- Feeling hot
- Making more saliva than usual (hypersalivation)
- Thirst
- Difficulty in concentrating (cognitive impairment)
- Memory problems
- Sleep disturbances
- Mood changes, crying or irritability.

Luckily, nobody seems to get them all. Researchers report that people generally have two or more of these symptoms, and the maximum number that one person gets is about seven.[3]

Yawning can be uncontrollable and frequent and, once you're aware of it, most people find this one quite easy to notice. You may need to be on the lookout for the others. Try and spot these clues, like a 'migraine detective'.

Keeping a migraine diary can help you notice when you're having premonitory symptoms of an attack. At first you'll be looking back to the days preceding the more obvious symptoms of aura or headache, but you may soon be able to spot premonitory symptoms as they happen, allowing you to treat your attack earlier and more effectively. Think about the snowball analogy: if you pick a snowball up and hold it in your hands while it's still small, it won't take long for it to melt away. Early intervention can make a huge difference to the impact that migraine has on your life.

Phase 2 – aura

The **aura phase** only occurs in about 25 per cent of people with migraine. It seems to be slightly more common among men. Neurochemicals carry messages around the body and brain and work by altering electrical charges on cells. It is thought aura is caused by so-called **cortical spreading depression** (CSD), where electrical signals flow in waves across the brain. Researchers are not certain yet why this causes the wide range of symptoms that people with aura describe, or why it doesn't cause aura in everyone with migraine.

> **Migraine without aura – the official definition**[4]
> Remember, about three in four people with migraine do not have aura. You have migraine without aura if:
>
> 1. Your headache lasts for four to seventy-two hours untreated (or treated unsuccessfully).
> 2. Your headache is characterized by at least two of the following:
>   • It's on one side.
>   • It has a pulsating quality.
>   • The pain is moderate to severe.

3. Your headache causes you to avoid routine physical activities like walking or climbing the stairs.
4. During the headache you had at least one of the following:
   - Nausea or vomiting
   - Sensitivity to light (photophobia) or sensitivity to sounds (phonophobia).
5. You have had least five attacks like this and they cannot be attributed to any other disorder.

The aura itself is a set of neurological symptoms that come and go, usually within the hour before the headache starts. Rarely, the aura and the headache start almost simultaneously. Aura symptoms may change in frequency over the course of your life. They may occur in youth and then disappear in adulthood, or vice versa. Some women get their first-ever aura attack during pregnancy.

Aura most commonly occurs as visual changes, with about 98 per cent of people who get aura describing a visual disturbance of some sort.[5] It can also be experienced as other sensory disturbances (in about 36 per cent of cases), language problems (about 10 per cent), dizziness (as in vestibular migraine) or motor weakness, where temporary paralysis of the muscles occurs (as in hemiplegic migraine).

Visual disturbances may be perceived in many different forms. In 2019 a group of researchers reviewed numerous studies on visual aura and compiled a list of twenty-five different 'elementary visual symptoms', including seeing zigzagged or jagged lines, flashes of bright light, foggy or blurred vision, blind spots (scotomata), black dots, visual snow and 'like looking through heat waves or water'.[6]

Some of the more unusual visual disturbances have rather beautiful-sounding names. They include 'hemianopsia' (half of the visual field is gone), 'metamorphopsia' (straight lines on a grid seem curvy) and 'oscillopsia' (objects around the person seem to jiggle around and move, even when they are still). 'Teichopsia' is the name given to a scintillating blind spot, which is basically two aura symptoms together – a gradual spreading of flashing, zigzagged light from the centre of the vision towards the periphery.

Distortions of vision can also occur, with things seeming to be further away than they really are. One of my patients described it to me as 'like looking down binoculars the wrong way round'. A less commonly described aura involves complex hallucinations where the person sees something that is not present, like a person or animal. Lewis Carroll, the author of *Alice in Wonderland*, had migraine attacks, according to his diaries. It has been suggested that visual aura may have inspired some of the fanciful scenes and characters in his stories, but this may just be neuromythology.[7]

It's important to identify aura in patients with migraine because this is associated with irregular, rapid heartbeats (atrial fibrillation), a condition that increases the risk of stroke, which is potentially life-threatening.[8] Women on oestrogen-containing contraceptive methods are potentially more at risk of stroke if they have aura.

Symptoms you might notice in the aura phase
Remember, only about one in four people with

migraine gets aura. Symptoms usually come and go within an hour:

- Visual disturbances
- Auditory hallucinations
- Smell hallucinations (phantosmias)
- Tingling sensations (paraesthesiae) or numbness
- Hearing reduction
- Weakness of the muscles on one side of the face or body
- Hiccups
- Chills
- Skin sensitivity
- Increased urination
- Neck pain
- Mood swings and irritability
- Fatigue and sleepiness.

Other types of aura are much rarer. Language issues can make life difficult if aura strikes while a person is at work. Transient aphasia can occur, where the person can't find their words – whether writing or speaking. They may know the right words, but mumble or sound garbled as they try to get them out. This once happened to a reporter presenting live at the Grammy Awards.

Some people with migraine with aura have described having auditory hallucinations. These can include the sound of human voices, music playing or repetitive beeping. These sounds are different from ringing in the ears (tinnitus). Such hallucinations are rare in migraine and can be caused by other conditions, so it is always best to get them investigated if you have them.

Olfactory hallucinations involve smells that are not there. Although these are not currently considered to be aura, they do seem to occur during this phase. People have described smelling unpleasant things: burning, smoke, gas, sulphur, rotten meat or metallic smells. Sometimes the smell can be more pleasant: melon, jasmine or vanilla.

Fortunately, by the nature of aura, all these disturbances are temporary and resolve fully by the end of the migraine attack.

I think of aura as the snowball gaining momentum and size. It's still not so big and fast-moving as to be very hard to stop. The snowball is somewhat powdery and lightly packed, and easy to squash. Taking medication at this stage might help to stop your gathering migraine in its tracks.

Phase 3 – headache

Next comes the **headache phase** that many people generally associate with having migraine. There is no doubt that this phase can be severe and disabling. The pain is often described as throbbing or pulsating. It may start anywhere on the head and move during an attack. Although classically described as one-sided, which gave migraine its name (the second-century CE Roman-Greek physician Galen called it *hemi-crania*, for pain affecting half the head[9]), it can be on both sides or can travel over the head. It can also be felt in the face, neck or shoulders.

The headache typically lasts from three to seventy-two

Premonition and aura
A tiny snowball, easily squashed with lifestyle changes, awareness and a rescue plan

Headache onset
A migraine attack rolling and gathering momentum – with quick, effective treatment, it can still be stopped

Headache without treatment
Digestion has slowed, making it much harder to absorb painkillers – so the attack keeps rolling and becoming more powerful until it settles naturally

Hangover
Migraine attack symptoms gradually melt away

Your migraine attack builds up, like a snowball rolling down a mountain

hours, often resolving in a shorter time in children than in adults. It may change from attack to attack, with some headaches being relatively mild and others very severe. This is often when nausea or vomiting strikes, and this may be extreme. Many people report increased sensitivity to light, sounds and smells. The skin on the scalp may become painful to touch. I have patients who can't put their hair up in a ponytail or even brush it when they have a headache. This heightened sensitivity to normal touch (allodynia) occurs especially in people with chronic migraine. A sensitivity to movement can make doing simple, everyday tasks of daily living, like emptying the dishwasher, unbearable. Often people in the midst of a bad headache phase will seek to be still and quiet in a darkened room. The headache can wake people up, though my patients sometimes say that sleeping helps lift the pain.

I think of this phase as the snowball gathering great momentum as it rushes down a mountain, growing firmer, bigger and more powerful.

Taking medication early in the headache phase is crucial. Leaving it too late – thinking that you'll delay taking a pain-killer until the headache is bad – can result in your medication being less effective or ineffective. If you get vomiting during the headache phase, it may be difficult even to keep the medicine down.

It is, however, possible for many people with migraine to shorten and reduce the severity of the headache phase. Strategies for this are discussed in Chapter 7.

Symptoms you may notice in the headache phase

- Headache – one-sided or both sides
- Pain in the face, neck or shoulders – again, one-sided or both sides
- Nausea or vomiting
- Increased sensitivity to light (photophobia), sounds (phonophobia), smells and movement
- Skin sensitivity (allodynia), particularly on the scalp
- Nasal congestion
- Abdominal pain
- Irritability.

Phase 4 – hangover

The fourth migraine phase is officially called the **postdromal phase**, but people with migraine often call it the 'hangover' because many of the symptoms mimic those you might feel after a heavy night out. A migraine hangover lasts from the time the headache finally goes until the person feels completely back to normal. This may be a couple of days. Some people find it quite disabling. It occurs in at least 80 per cent of attacks.[10]

Hangover symptoms often take about one to two days to resolve, no matter how severe the headache has been or what medication the person has taken. Most people – up to 88 per cent in one study[11] – report feeling drained. More than half have difficulty with concentration. About 42 per cent say their stiff neck continues from the headache phase. Light and sound sensitivities can remain troublesome, and nausea can persist too.

Some also notice the return of premonitory symptoms. It seems likely that brain changes which cause these symptoms to start in the first phase continue through aura and headache into the hangover. People recovering from migraine headache often under-report their hangover symptoms, especially neck stiffness and light and sound sensitivities. This may be because they are so relieved the headache is going that they don't find the lingering symptoms noteworthy.

Returning to my snowball analogy, this is when the snowball melts away. It doesn't disappear quickly, but gradually reduces, with its impact lessening, until it's gone.

<u>**Symptoms you may notice in the**</u>
<u>**hangover phase**</u>

- **Weakness and lethargy**
- **Skin looking pale (pallor)**
- **Sleepiness**
- **Difficulties with thinking and problem-solving**
  (cognitive impairment)
- **Nausea**
- **Food cravings**
- **Thirst**
- **Tingling (paraesthesia)**
- **Eye pain**
- **Visual disturbances**

Once the migraine attack has settled completely, the person enters what is sometimes called the **interictal phase**. Your symptoms have fully resolved and you're feeling back to normal – what I call 'crystal-clear' days. In my clinic I ask patients to count up these days too, both to savour them and to get a better understanding of the frequency of their attacks.

Sadly, for too many people the snowball of migraine will start to roll again. In those with chronic migraine or medication-overuse headache, there may be very few crystal-clear days each month, and daily activities such as working, studying and socializing become a struggle.

Is it worth searching for triggers?

When my patients and I begin to discuss a plan for managing their migraine, they are understandably hoping to find one thing they might do, or stop doing, to make their attacks cease. Unfortunately it's not that simple. It is more helpful to think of triggers adding together to irritate the brain, pushing its sensitivity towards a threshold. Once the threshold is breached, a migraine attack starts to roll.

Some researchers think nerve cells in a migraine brain are not as good at generating energy as they need to be. When these cells experience a drop in energy, they are more easily overloaded by sensory inputs. When this happens in the hypothalamus and brainstem, it leads to activation of the **trigeminovascular system**, a network of nerves in the brain that communicates pain signals, and this sets a migraine attack rolling.[12]

As we have seen, the first, premonitory phase of a migraine attack can start up to seventy-two hours before the aura or headache. This is when the migraine brain first begins to react

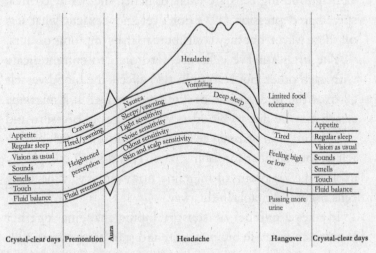

The phases of a migraine attack.
Adapted with permission of the National Migraine Centre, London.

to sensory overload. Because many people don't realize they are in the premonitory phase, they may confuse early symptoms of an attack with what's triggering the attack.

Sensory inputs are registered by the body, with your nerves sending signals back to nerve cells in the brain, literally exciting them. The electrical signals trigger the production of neurochemicals and hormones like serotonin.[13] The electrical charge within groups of excited cells also changes, with the charge inside each cell becoming more positive compared to the charge outside it.

In talking about the aura phase, I mentioned the phenomenon of cortical spreading depression (CSD). In people with migraine, the charge in nerve cells alters in waves that roll over the brain's surface (cortex), with a group of cells being excited and then quieting (and becoming more negative in charge) as neighbouring cells are excited, hence the name 'cortical spreading depression'.[14] We don't yet know exactly what sets off these waves, but they contribute to the symptoms of aura.

The brain's nerve cells use serotonin to communicate with each other, but serotonin also affects the blood vessels all over the body. Some of the pain we feel in a migraine attack may be due to blood-vessel changes in pressure and to inflammation of brain cells (neurogenic inflammation)[15] – felt as that familiar throbbing pain. This doesn't completely explain the symptoms of migraine, however, or why the nerve cells become irritable in this way.

It takes a number of sensory inputs changing together to push an irritable brain too far and start these waves rolling. People may report weather changes, food cravings and poor sleep as triggers, but these may simply be noticed more intensely during the first or second phase of a migraine attack that is under way. The brain is already hyper-sensitized.

You may not find a clear pattern, even if you try to note down possible triggers. Some triggers may always cause an attack while others only do so occasionally.

In essence, what triggers a migraine attack is 'change'. For this reason, in my experience it's less important to pinpoint specific triggers and more important to establish a routine that helps you reduce change by managing the things you can control.

Changes you can and can't control

So where does change commonly come into our lives?

- **Stress**: This is possibly the factor most commonly cited as an attack trigger in my clinic, and a great deal of research supports this view.[16] Interestingly, often a *reduction* in stress can lead to weekend or 'let-down' headaches. Stress hormones such as cortisol are also released and fluctuate when you're excited or emotional. Patients who have been told their migraine attacks are 'probably just because you are stressed' tend to find this unhelpful and may feel as though their symptoms are being dismissed. Plus, it's not that simple to 'switch off' stress.
- **Sleep**: Good sleep patterns are important for people with migraine. Missing sleep, broken sleep and prolonged, extra hours of sleep can all trigger an attack.
- **Sex hormones**: Many women with migraine identify a pattern of attacks around the time of their period. This is

due to fluctuations in the sex hormone oestrogen during the menstrual cycle. Some women have worsening symptoms around the menopause as their oestrogen levels decrease.

- **Growth hormones**: Hormones may also trigger attacks in teenagers. The pituitary gland produces more growth hormone during growth spurts. Levels of testosterone in boys and oestrogen in girls also change during puberty. But a teenager's migraine attacks can also be started by other changing factors. Teenagers have different sleep patterns and dietary habits, and a host of other stresses and excitements.

- **Food**: Many people with migraine feel sure they have identified specific dietary triggers for their attacks. The classic, oft-blamed culprit is chocolate, but craving chocolate is probably a prodromal symptom. There are lots of books offering 'migraine diets' and long lists on the internet of foods to exclude in order to 'heal' your brain. True food triggers are actually rare. Researchers have tried to look into whether there are any useful, menu-based strategies for people with migraine, but none have found conclusive, reproducible evidence that elimination of any particular food, or following any specific diet, will work for everybody. If, however, you have observed that eating a particular food always triggers an attack for you, then it makes sense to avoid it. Endlessly searching for a blame-worthy 'trigger food' is probably not worthwhile, though, and may lead to poor nutrition if you try to follow one of the extreme elimination diets. What is more important is regulating your blood-sugar levels so that you aren't experiencing a roller-coaster of ups and downs in one day.

- **Drink**: About one-third of people with migraine find that alcohol is a trigger for them,[17] and in my clinic I've had many patients stop drinking alcohol altogether, saying, 'It's just not worth it.' However, drinking alcohol doesn't have a consistent effect, and the type of alcohol leading to an attack may vary from person to person and over time. If alcohol is a trigger, it can have effects rapidly, within three hours of drinking; or rather more slowly, giving a headache several hours afterwards, like a classic hangover. Alcohol can also cause blood glucose to fall, can lead to dehydration, impair the quality of a person's sleep and be used as a stress reliever or for a celebration where excitement levels are high. For some people, caffeine may be the offender. Dehydration may trigger attacks too. All of these factors may make migraine more likely.
- **Weather**: Weather sensitivity is reported by some people as a trigger, and there have been several studies on the link between weather and migraine. Factors like humidity, temperature and atmospheric pressure changes have been investigated, with mixed results.[18] It seems that a drop in barometric pressure leading to more changeable, rainy weather is more likely to bother people than other weather factors.[19] Thundery weather is associated with low pressure, and some researchers have found that more migraine attacks appear to happen on days when lightning occurs. They suggest this may be due to an electromagnetic effect.[20] They did not find any evidence of technical sources, such as power lines or mobile phones, causing migraine.
- **Lights, patterns and seasons**: It is well known that people with migraine get an aversion to bright light

(photophobia), especially during attacks. Now researchers are looking into several questions: Can light trigger attacks? Is light sensitivity a premonitory symptom? And are people with migraine sensitive to light all the time, even when they are between attacks? Curiously, exposing people with migraine to bright, flashing light in laboratory settings does not trigger an attack, even in those who think light is a trigger for them. In Norway, during the time of year when the sun never sets, researchers found that the frequency of migraine attacks increased by about 12 per cent.[21] Between attacks, some people with migraine are more sensitive to patterns, especially stripes and highly contrasting colours. I've had patients who find it difficult to look at light coming through Venetian blinds, at grids or at spotted or striped clothing.

- **Odours**: A sensitivity to odours (osmophobia) is a symptom in migraine attacks that is often described as a trigger too. Just the whiff of an offending smell can quickly start an attack rolling. Sitting on the bus next to a person doused in their favourite perfume can trigger a migraine attack within ten minutes. It's really helpful for a person with this trigger when work colleagues are considerate and avoid wearing strong fragrances or eating strong-smelling foods. This too seems to be a sensitivity that exists between attacks.

- **Exercise and physical activity**: Certain types of exercise can trigger an attack, a topic that we'll explore in more detail in Chapter 4. I have also heard from patients who have tried massage or other physical therapies on their neck and shoulders and this has aggravated rather than helped their migraine. Others find massage helpful, however.

It may be that there are subsets of people with migraine who react to certain triggers, while others do not. Once again we return to the idea that triggers add up. It takes several triggering factors accumulating for an attack to start in a susceptible individual. But if you have identified something that always gives you an attack, it makes sense to avoid it, wherever possible.

Some headache specialists believe learning to 'cope' with triggers, rather than avoiding them altogether, may be a better approach.[22] They suggest that complete avoidance may heighten a person's sensitivity. For example, people who wear sunglasses all the time may become more sensitive to light. The science is not clear on this, however.

Routine can minimize the chance that your triggers will add together and start the snowball of a migraine attack rolling. Similarly, limiting change in your daily life may reduce your migraine frequency. In my clinic I point to the areas where we have the most control: how regularly and what we eat; how and what we do for exercise; and when we sleep. We'll look at each of these over the next three chapters, before turning to how we respond to stress – the most common trigger, and perhaps the one we most need to reduce.

3. When and What You Eat

You may have searched, perhaps with frustration, for that elusive diet that might finally solve your migraine. Avoiding certain foods, giving up alcohol and cutting back on caffeine are all strategies my patients have explored. Many have tried adding herbal products or supplements to their regime. Finding a recipe for success in this way takes a lot of effort – and could cost you a great deal of money!

There's no doubt that your brain and your gut are closely linked, so finding a healthy, balanced approach to diet and nutrition will help you keep your brain healthy too. In this chapter we'll review some dietary changes that people have found helpful and will flag up what to avoid and what not to bother with.

Watching your blood-sugar levels

The glycaemic index (GI) is a measure of the effect that foods have on blood-sugar (glucose) levels. Foods with a high GI cause your blood glucose to rise rapidly, triggering the release of insulin from your pancreas (if your pancreas is healthy). This rush of insulin lowers blood-glucose levels by tucking the glucose away as fat, predominantly in your fat cells and liver. If this happens repeatedly, your cells may become resistant to the effects of insulin, so the pancreas has to make more to see the same reduction in your blood glucose.

Low-GI foods, sometimes called 'slow-release energy foods', cause a slower rise in blood sugar and more sustained energy release to fuel your body. Reducing fluctuations in blood-glucose levels does seem to help some people avoid migraine attacks.[1] There appears to be less inflammation in people following a low-GI diet too.

Why this happens isn't clear. Researchers have observed that some people with migraine have higher-than-average insulin levels in their blood and insulin resistance, although it is not known yet if this is part of the cause of migraine or a coincidence.[2] For example, higher levels of neurochemicals linked with inflammation and pain pathways are found in some people who are obese. Regardless, a low-GI diet might help you reduce your migraine attacks.

It is not always easy to guess the GI index for a specific food, but there are numerous tables available. Don't assume everything that's sweet scores a high GI. The table overleaf illustrates just how tricky it can be guessing these scores. With more familiarity, you'll get a sense of which foods are likely to be low GI and which high GI. As a simple guide, slower-release energy foods to aim for include vegetables, high-fibre foods like wholegrains, pulses and legumes, and some fruits like berries.

Your blood-glucose levels will fall if you have an early-evening meal and eat nothing again until a late breakfast, or if you have a long gap between meals or exercise vigorously. Some people with migraine report that prolonged periods of not eating (fasting) trigger an attack. Varying blood-glucose levels may especially affect active children.

For these reasons, I recommend that people with migraine:

Food	GI
Jacket potato	111
Glucose (standard)	100
Cornflakes	81
Watermelon (raw)	76
White bread	75
Popcorn	65
Chips/French fries	63
Soft/fizzy drink	59
Porridge	55
Wholegrain bread	53
Orange juice	50
Milk chocolate	43
Strawberries	41
Carrots (boiled)	39
Full-fat milk	39
Brussels sprouts	32
Chickpeas	28
Dark chocolate	23
Cherries	20
Broccoli	10

Some foods and their approximate glycaemic-index (GI) value[3]

- Avoid skipping meals.
- Have something to eat every three to four hours.
- Try a bedtime snack of low-GI, slow-release energy foods.

One study of people with migraine on a low-GI diet found that the frequency and intensity of their headaches reduced significantly after three months. Some of my patients who have taken a low-GI approach to their diet say that not only has the frequency of their migraine attacks lessened, but they have also lost weight. They report having more energy and generally feeling better too.

Watching your carbs intake

In recent years two diets have received a great deal of attention for their potential to reduce inflammation and improve health: the ketogenic diet and a modified version of the Atkins diet.[4]

The **ketogenic diet** has been used for the treatment of conditions like epilepsy and diabetes and recently there has been interest in trying it for migraine.[5] The goal is to reduce the carbohydrates in your diet to such an extent that your body starts to use your stored fat as fuel, converting it into what are called 'ketone bodies', which are thought to have an anti-inflammatory effect. The diet may work by acting on the mitochondria (tiny organelles inside cells that produce energy for our bodies). It may also protect nerve cells and regulate how brain cells are excited by inputs. To follow a ketogenic diet, you must carefully weigh and log foods to monitor the proportion of carbohydrates, proteins and fat in everything you eat. It's easy to slip into eating more carbs than the diet recommends. It's also important to keep well hydrated if you try this diet. Some people on a ketogenic diet fast, eating supper no later than 7 p.m. and delaying breakfast until around noon the next day. This may not suit your migrainous brain. The change from running the body's engine on carbs to running it on ketones also causes some people to feel flu-like symptoms initially.

The **modified Atkins diet** is slightly less restrictive than the ketogenic diet and some people find it easier to follow. Weight loss often occurs on both diets, sometimes quite rapidly.

If you decide to try one of these diets, first consult a healthcare professional experienced in dietary and nutritional advice, who will make sure the diet is suitable for you and will help you work out how best to follow it.

Watching your weight

Obesity has been associated with many health issues, and so researchers have investigated whether it contributes to worsening migraine. The evidence is somewhat mixed, but points to a connection. There seems to be a higher risk of episodic migraine turning into chronic migraine if a person is obese.[6] Being obese is also associated with more severe pain and more frequent attacks.[7] Metabolic syndrome, a pre-diabetic condition, is possibly associated with more migraine too.[8] This may be due to the release of inflammatory chemicals from fatty tissue. There is certainly a link between obesity and a different type of primary headache called idiopathic intracranial hypertension (IIH), where pressure in the brain increases for an unknown reason (see Chapter 13).[9]

For those who are obese, losing weight is rarely as 'simple' as eating less and exercising more, since a range of genetic, social and environmental factors help to shape people's weight. Further, eating less and exercising more may trigger attacks in people with migraine. So while losing weight through diet and exercise may be possible, other weight-loss strategies might be considered. Weight-loss or bariatric surgery (which restricts your stomach so that you feel full sooner, changing your appetite and metabolism) has been found to help reduce attacks, and may even be better at lessening headache than other weight-loss methods.[10]

More research is needed to work out how weight is related to migraine and the best way to help people with migraine who want to reduce their weight.

Watching your fat intake

You may have heard that saturated fats are best avoided. Polyunsaturated fats, like omega-3 and omega-6, have been studied too, and the ratio of omega-3 to omega-6 seems to be most important for our health.[11]

Many people have too much omega-6 in their diet. This polyunsaturated fat occurs in corn and vegetable oils found in many processed foods, including crisps, cakes, fried and cured meats. Omega-3 is plentiful in oily fish like salmon, flaxseeds, kidney beans, mangoes, spinach and even lettuce. Some foods high in omega-6, like walnuts, also contain omega-3 and are a bit healthier.

Studies that have looked at low-fat diets for people with migraine have found that it's probably the type of fat you eat, rather than the amount, that is key. People eating diets high in omega-3 and lower in omega-6 seem to have fewer headaches than those who simply reduce their omega-6 intake. Adding nanocurcumin – a form of curcumin found in the spice turmeric – to omega-3-rich meals may help too.

Exclusion diets

We began this chapter by looking at more holistic diets because, as I mentioned in Chapter 2, when it comes to managing migraine, it's rarely necessary to exclude one, two or even a handful of things from your diet.

To start to work out which food – if any – is triggering your attacks, you would need to eliminate the suspected food completely from your diet for at least a month (the elimination phase) and then return to eating it (the provocation phase) and see what happens. If your headaches disappear, only to return when the food is eaten again, then your answer is clear. Many people in my clinic have tried this process. A few have successfully identified a problem food. More have not. Even chocolate, with its bad reputation for triggering migraine, has not been proven to trigger attacks. The latest thinking is that cravings for chocolate and some other foods are symptoms of the premonitory phase of a migraine attack.[12]

Migraine is a complex condition with many interacting variables. Researchers looking at possible food intolerances have tested the blood of patients for immunoglobulin G (IgG) antibodies against certain foods, to see if they could identify people's food triggers. Our immune system produces antibodies to fight infection by viruses or bacteria but also, not so usefully, sometimes against things that should be harmless, such as certain foods. The people in the study said they noticed an improvement in the number of headaches they experienced when they stopped eating the foods flagged by the antibody test. The improvement seemed to be especially noticed by people who also had irritable bowel syndrome (IBS). The researchers concluded that the blood test they used, called an ELISA blood test, could be useful to help people with migraine decide which foods they might avoid.[13] More research in this area would be helpful.

So let's turn to some specific things you may have considered excluding from your diet.

- **Histamine**: A neurochemical implicated in hay fever and allergies, histamine is found in some foodstuffs, including fermented foods such as alcohol and yoghurt, cured meats, shellfish, dried fruits, avocados and spinach. Some patients ask me about avoiding it in their diet.

  There are four receptors in the body for histamine, called, imaginatively, H_1, H_2, H_3 and H_4. Over-the-counter antihistamine tablets work on H_1 to block the action of histamine and stop your runny nose and sneezing.

  Histamine in relation to migraine is more complex. There is currently no clear evidence that drugs which block the H_1, H_2 or H_4 receptors reduce migraine. These receptors don't appear to be found in the brain. In contrast, the H_3 receptor is found in the brain and across the nervous system. Research on the H_3 receptor, and the development of medications to act on it, is promising but needs more investigation.

  So does this mean you should exclude histamine-containing foods from your diet? The only study on this dates back to 1993[14] and required a very restrictive diet that could result in nutritional deficiencies, if not

47

supervised by an expert. If you have a lot of allergies, such as chronic hives (urticaria), it may be helpful.

- **Tyramine**: This is another neurochemical reported to be a migraine trigger. It is found in food as it ages, which is why aged cheeses, pickles, smoked and processed meats, sourdough bread, other fermented foods and red wine have gained a reputation as triggers. Some people exclude dairy products to lower their intake of these compounds. It's not clear how important these compounds are, and there have been few studies since the 1990s on their role in migraine. As tyramine is widely found in foods, eliminating it can be extremely difficult.

- **Gluten**: This is found in wheat, barley, rye and, to some extent, oats. In people with coeliac disease, eating the protein gliadin, which occurs in our diet as gluten, causes problems. Coeliac disease is diagnosed by blood tests and biopsy. Once diagnosed, a person with coeliac disease should follow a lifelong, strict gluten-free diet.

    Coeliac disease is a condition where genetic factors seem to make people more susceptible to migraine, and people with headache have an increased prevalence of coeliac disease.[15] The headaches reported by people with coeliac disease are predominantly migraine, so this is one condition linked with headache that does benefit from a strict gluten-free diet.

    If you have a family history of coeliac disease, or suspect you may have it because of other symptoms, it is important to get a blood test before starting a gluten-free diet. If you have already cut out gluten for a while, the test may be falsely negative.

- **Caffeine**: Who among us can say we have never had any caffeine in our lives? Not many, I'm guessing. Worldwide about 80 per cent of adults have a caffeinated drink *every* day.[16] This is one of humanity's favourite mood-altering, fatigue-battling drugs. It is present naturally in coffee, tea, cocoa and kola-nut plants, but it is also found in nearly sixty other different plant species. It's increasingly being added to soft drinks. There is even caffeinated bottled water! Caffeine seems to enhance the effects of simple painkillers such as aspirin, paracetamol and ibuprofen, and it often appears among the ingredients of combination painkillers on sale in shops and advertised as being helpful for migraine. However, its effect on migraine is complicated.[17]

  Caffeine works by blocking the action of adenosine, an important chemical that helps us get off to sleep. Even having a low dose of caffeine regularly seems to aggravate sleep disruption and can worsen insomnia. It is not so useful as a painkiller on its own, but it helps painkillers do their job, which is why it is sometimes called an 'analgesic adjuvant'. I've had patients describe treating their migraine attacks successfully with painkillers and a can of Coca-Cola.

  One of the ways caffeine helps in migraine is by improving the emptying of the stomach. When a migraine attack is starting, your gut slows down (gastric stasis). This can lead to nausea and sometimes vomiting but also, importantly, it slows down the absorption of painkillers. Caffeine seems to counteract this.

  If you take too much caffeine too often, you may increase the risk of your episodic migraine attacks turning into chronic migraine. You could also increase the risk of developing medication-overuse headache. Reducing caffeine gradually until it's been removed from the diet has been helpful for some people with migraine, especially those with vestibular migraine, where the main symptom is dizziness (see Chapter 12). Suddenly withdrawing caffeine may cause headaches, however. This may be one contributory factor to weekend migraine attacks.

I recommend using caffeine in moderation. Having one or two cups of coffee in the morning and none after 1 p.m. might be a good rule of thumb. A dose of 130mg

Food or drink	Serving size	Caffeine content
Starbucks – regular	474ml (16 fl. oz)	259mg
Coffee – brewed	237ml (8 fl. oz)	70–140mg (average 95mg)
Espresso – 1 shot	30–50ml (2 fl. oz)	63–120mg
Red Bull	245 ml (8.3 fl. oz)	75–80mg
Tea – brewed black	237ml (8 fl. oz)	50–60mg
Coca-Cola – 1 can	355 ml (12 fl. oz)	45mg
Green tea	237ml (8 fl. oz)	28mg
Chocolate bar	28g (1 oz)	15mg
Decaf coffee – brewed	237ml (8 fl. oz)	3–6mg
Rooibos tea	237mg (8 fl. oz)	0mg

Just how much caffeine are you getting?

Doses will vary in brewed drinks like tea and coffee, depending on how you make your cuppa and the type of leaf or bean.

High-caffeine energy drinks have been associated with side-effects such as seizures, stroke and, rarely, even death. Remember: caffeine is a powerful psychoactive drug.

seems to be the optimal amount for helping migraine in people who have not developed a tolerance to it from frequent use.

'Have you been drinking enough water?'

This question is frequently thrown at people with migraine. Wouldn't it be lovely if an extra glass or two was the answer to migraine? But although hydration is frequently quoted as a factor in migraine attacks, there is nothing in the medical literature proving that water deprivation causes any sort of headache. Plus, we are not really sure how much water is enough and, of course, the amount you need each day will vary, depending on the ambient temperature and humidity, and your activity levels, diet and the functioning of your kidneys and bowel. Medications and alcohol can also affect the balance of water in your body.

Drinking a few more glasses of water a day is a simple and cheap thing to do, so try seeing if it helps you. If drinking more water helps your migraine, go ahead. Don't overdo it, though. Drinking excessive amounts of water is not a good idea and can even be harmful.

Complementary nutritional therapies

An increasing number of the people I see in my clinic are trying products available over the counter in health-food shops and pharmacies, or from the internet, to try and reduce their migraine symptoms. These may be vitamins, mineral supplements or herbal remedies. It's vital that you give your doctor or headache specialist the whole picture of what you take, including supplements, as they can interact with other medications.

Nutraceuticals

The disturbance of energy production in brain cells may play an important part in generating migraine attacks, which has led to increasing interest in how taking food supplements called **nutraceuticals** might help regulate these metabolic changes.

Three particular food nutraceutical supplements have some evidence of benefit for people with migraine: magnesium, riboflavin and coenzyme Q10.[18] The target doses for these supplements are high. I recommend starting with a low dose and increasing slowly. If you decide to try one, two or all three, they each need to be taken for at least three months before you can tell if they are helping. In many countries, including the UK, they are not usually available on prescription, so cost may be a factor in your decision.

- **Magnesium**: This is a hugely important mineral, needed in more than 300 essential chemical reactions in the body. Typical blood tests for magnesium measure what is called 'extracellular' or serum levels of magnesium, which accounts for only about 1 per cent of the magnesium in your body. When researchers have looked at 'intracellular' magnesium inside the red blood cells – a better measure of magnesium status – they have found that people with migraine have low magnesium levels, especially so among women with menstrually related migraine, it seems (see Chapter 9).[19] In some studies magnesium has been given, in high doses (usually 600mg a day of magnesium citrate), for three months to see if this might reduce attacks, with promising results.[20] Other magnesium salts – for example, magnesium malate and magnesium glycinate – are available and may be as effective. Magnesium is usually safe and well tolerated, but some people who take it by mouth have soft stools or diarrhoea (one of the symptoms of low magnesium is constipation). Changing the type you take may settle this. Check with your doctor before you start magnesium, especially if you have a history of kidney or liver problems.

- **Riboflavin (vitamin B2):** This is another vitamin involved in energy production in the mitochondria of our cells. There is some evidence that this process is deficient in the cells of people with migraine. A high dose of 400mg a day has been found to be well tolerated and helpful for preventing migraine attacks in adults. In children the picture is not quite so clear, but riboflavin may also be helpful. Be warned, though: this vitamin colours the urine a strong yellow colour. It's not harmful – but it can be alarming if you aren't expecting it!

- **Coenzyme Q10:** This nutraceutical is also thought to act on the parts of our cells responsible for energy production. Doses of 100mg three times a day, used for at least three months, have been found to reduce migraine frequency in some adults.[21]

- **Vitamin D:** This important supplement is actually not a vitamin, but a hormone. It helps to increase your body's absorption of minerals like calcium and phosphorus. It is largely made by the action of sunlight on your skin and

is commonly low in people who are living at higher lati-
tudes, like the UK, with very short winter days. It is also
often low in those who have darker skin pigmentation or
who avoid sun exposure, regularly use high-factor sun-
screen or rarely go outside during daylight hours – for
example, night-shift workers. Many studies have found
a low vitamin D level in people with migraine and have
tried to establish if this simply comes down to low
vitamin D levels being a common issue or if migraine
is aggravated by low vitamin D.[22] The answer is still
not known, but since vitamin D is important for good
immunity, regulating calcium, supporting insulin metabolism and, of course, maintaining strong bones and teeth,
it's a good idea to make sure your vitamin D levels are
optimized. Your doctor can order a blood test to check
your levels, or advise on a suitable dose to take on a
weekly or daily basis.

Herbal remedies

People sometimes think herbal remedies are healthier or safer
because they are 'natural'. This is not always the case. It's often
difficult to assess the effect of herbal remedies because there is
great variability in the formulations, doses and proportions of
active ingredients from producer to producer. Some may have
potentially toxic components too, or may interact with medications that you take. Rigorous safety testing is often not done
or is unavailable, and effective doses and the duration of treatment are hard to specify with any certainty. Keep in mind that
herbal remedies are basically drugs and cause pharmacological

effects in the body, so you should always tell your doctor or headache specialist about any herbal remedy you are considering or already taking.

Two herbal remedies are often mentioned for treating migraine: feverfew and butterbur. One *may* sometimes be safe. The other is not.

- **Feverfew** (*Tanacetum parthenium*): This herb has been used for migraine for centuries. Its active ingredient, a chemical called parthenolide, acts on the central nervous system. Parthenolide has been studied, and the consensus seems to be that it is well tolerated and may help some adults prevent attacks, although no specific dose has been specified. It can have side-effects of gastrointestinal upset and mouth ulcers. Long-term use has been associated with something called 'post-feverfew' syndrome – anxiety, insomnia, muscle and joint stiffness and even headache. It should never be used during pregnancy.

- **Butterbur** (*Petasites hybridus*): This herb was used for migraine prevention for centuries. However, increasing concerns about the damage it causes to the liver mean that doctors now advise that people do *not* take it. The problem is a group of chemicals called pyrrolizidine alkaloids that are toxic to the liver. It is banned in some European countries because of this.

The gut–brain axis

It's amazing to think of all the ways in which when – and what – you eat might help your migraine. The relationship between the brain and the gut is one that scientists are only beginning to fully understand.

We know that the brain and the gut communicate directly with each other partly by way of the vagus nerve and neuro-chemical signals. This system has been dubbed the **gut–brain axis**.[23] How the gut and brain interact is a function of many different factors, including the level of your stress hormones and your nutritional intake. Proteins made by nerve cells (neuro-peptides) and other inflammatory mediators like histamine are also known to be involved. And it seems that the billions of bacteria that thrive in our gut environment, our **microbiome**, are crucially important too.

These colonies of bacteria help to maintain a healthy immune system and regulate the metabolism of glucose. A person with less diverse bacteria in their gut seems to have an increased risk of obesity. This is one of the contributory fac-tors that can make it difficult for an obese person to lose weight. A poor diet, often with a low dietary-fibre intake, and medica-tions like antibiotics and proton-pump inhibitor drugs – for example, omeprazole, which is commonly used to treat acid reflux and certain ulcers – can reduce the diversity and health of your microbiome. Increasing your dietary fibre and sup-plementing your diet with prebiotic foods and probiotic-rich fermented foods, live yoghurts or supplements may improve the health of your microbiome. Prebiotic foods contain a type of fibre that nourishes the helpful micro-organisms, known as probiotics, which are important for maintaining your micro-biome and gut health.

It is known that there is a link between migraine and certain gut disorders like IBS, inflammatory bowel disease (IBD) and coeliac disease. The bacterium *Helicobacter pylori*, which has been linked to duodenal ulcers, also appear to be more common in the gut of people with migraine.[24] But a lot of questions still remain to be answered about the microbiome and its relevance to migraine.

A diet for success?

Taking into consideration all the competing scientific evidence, it's clear that there is no single approach to diet or nutritional supplements that will work for everybody with migraine. Instead, people with migraine must make their own personal decisions about diet, based on observing their attacks, weighing up any other conditions (such as IBS or allergies) that they have, and conferring with their doctor or headache specialist about what to try. Some dietary strategies may work well for me, but not for you.

Avoid becoming overly obsessed with food diaries. They are rarely helpful. True food triggers are very consistent in producing a migraine attack. They are also much rarer than people think.

At the same time, based on the experience of countless patients, diet and nutrition – and particularly keeping a consistent schedule for meals – may prove to be one of the cornerstones of effective management of your migraine.

And it's important to note that our blood-sugar levels aren't affected solely by the food we eat. In the next chapter we'll look at how exercise and posture can affect the brain too.

Maria's story

Maria came to see me, complaining of having migraine attacks on fifteen to twenty days each month. She told me how miserable she felt. She was comforting herself by eating lots of sugary foods and drinking numerous fizzy drinks. We talked about the importance of timing meals and looking at trying to reduce those high-carbohydrate foods and drinks.

When she returned three months later, she came in smiling. She had stopped the fizzy drinks, added in more vegetables, protein and healthy fats, and was now only getting one migraine attack per month. She had also dropped two dress sizes! She was surprised and delighted at how easy it had been to make these changes and improve her migraine attacks.

Take note of the glycaemic index of the meals and snacks you're eating. Reducing spikes in blood-glucose levels can be a great help.

4. Exercising Body and Brain

Exercise is so beneficial for our general health it has been said that, if exercise were a drug, it would be prescribed for everyone. We should all move more and sit less. But is this old axiom true for migraine?

Well, it depends. It depends on how you exercise, how long you exercise and what type of exercise you do. Some types of exercise may help, while others may trigger an attack. In this chapter we'll explore this and look at the role of posture and the use of physical therapies like physiotherapy, osteopathy, ice packs and heat to help reduce the frequency or severity of attacks.

However you decide to bring these approaches into your life, keep in mind that an irritable brain doesn't like change. Get moving, but start slowly and increase any physical activity gradually.

How can exercise help?

You may have heard of, or even experienced, the phenomenon called a 'runner's high'. This is a sudden positive sensation of euphoria after certain types of extended physical exertion. The 'high' arrives after the release of two groups of chemicals – **endorphins** and **endocannabinoids** – which help relieve pain, stress and inflammation. Both chemical groups appear to play a role in migraine.

Endorphins are sometimes called the 'body's opioids'. When released by the body, they help reduce pain. Exercising regularly has been shown to increase levels of one endorphin, beta-endorphin, which blocks pain pathways in the body from being triggered. Beta-endorphin levels tend to be lower in people with migraine, especially those with chronic migraine.[1]

Endocannabinoids appear to work similarly to cannabinoids, the chemicals in cannabis. Levels of one endocannabinoid, anandamide (AEA), have also been found to be lower in people with migraine.[2] AEA is not released during low-intensity walking. It takes high-intensity or endurance running to activate release of this feel-good system. Endocannabinoids are higher in the morning and after a good restful night's sleep – a sound reason to get up and out into the daylight in the morning.

Studies have found that exercising might help to release more beta-endorphin and AEA in people with naturally lower levels.[3] Researchers have also looked at taking exercise to prevent migraine.[4] In one study, people with migraine were assigned to: 1) take a drug specifically prescribed for preventing migraine; or 2) follow a programme of relaxation and breathing exercises; or 3) exercise for forty minutes three times a week.[5] The groups who exercised or did breathing exercises had the same reduction in frequency of attacks over twelve weeks as those who took medication. Another study, this one of an aerobic endurance training programme building up to thirty minutes of jogging over a ten-week period, found that not only were people's migraine attacks reduced with exercise, but their attention and information-processing improved too.[6]

Of course exercise also helps build your energy levels, enhances feelings of well-being and mood, keeps your heart and blood pressure healthy and helps you sleep better. Cognitive functions, such as concentration, memory and problem-solving, may improve.[7] The positive feeling that you are lessening the impact of migraine – and living your life, despite migraine – may lift your spirits.

Many of my patients feel their migraine dominates what they do. Exercise helps them to take back some control.

Can exercise make migraine worse?

While exercise might help with your migraine, it doesn't help everyone. As we saw in Chapter 2, migraine pain can worsen when you move, and some people find that exercise triggers an attack. This may put you off exercising altogether. I have certainly had many adults and children in my clinic tell me they have had to stop or change the way they exercise because of their attacks. And there's no clear pattern to what sorts of exercise might trigger an attack. Running, lifting weights at the gym, playing football, ice-skating and ballet have all been cited as triggers by my patients.

There is some evidence that people with migraine tend to do less physical exercise between attacks. Some researchers link low physical-activity levels with more migraine attacks,[8] but this may be something of a 'chicken and egg' situation as to which came first. When researchers have looked into this, they have found that about 38 per cent of people with migraine report exercise as a trigger, with more than half saying they had to quit a sport that triggered it.[9] Neck pain seemed to be a predominant feature, as did the intensity of activity. High-intensity aerobic exercise, such as indoor cycling on a spin bike, appears to be more likely to start an attack rolling. Some people said that switching to lower-intensity activities enabled them to continue exercising.

Some researchers have suggested that people with migraine may have a problem with efficient energy metabolism in their cells. This may be why attacks are often associated with exercise. Others think changes in heart rate and blood pressure cause changes to the blood vessels in the brain, starting an attack. Another theory is that the hypothalamus – that small part of the brain which sets off the release of various hormones – is involved. Sleep patterns can change following intense exercise, and it could be that a neurochemical called hypocretin, which helps regulate our sleep and arousal and is tied to narcolepsy, may be a key factor. We aren't sure yet.

Another factor may be lactic acid. This is produced in muscles when you're exercising hard. A build-up of lactic acid is what gives you a 'stitch', or the burning sensation while you're exercising. It happens when the body switches from using oxygen (aerobic energy) to using glucose released from cells (anaerobic energy) because the energy you need outstrips your supply of oxygen. This is not dangerous, but it leads to higher levels of lactate in your blood and brain.

Blood levels of another pain chemical, calcitonin gene-related peptide (CGRP), have been shown to rise during exercise too. One study showed that athletes running a half-marathon had 1.5 times higher concentrations of CGRP in their blood after their run.[10] New medications to target CGRP are very exciting, as we'll see in Chapters 7 and 8.

But don't let this put you off exercising. Exercise benefits your brain and body in many ways. It's well worth taking the time to discover which types of exercise you like and then slowly building them up as a regular part of your routine. This will help keep you healthy while also reducing the chances of triggering an attack.

Once you decide on your exercise regime, pace yourself. Make sure you are well hydrated and have enough 'brain fuel' on board by having a light, easily digestible snack like oatcakes, a handful of nuts or a banana, before and afterwards. The migraine brain does not like being starved, and exercising uses up blood glucose more rapidly. It's also important to do warm-up and cool-down routines around your exercise.

Regular exercising at moderate intensity – just enough to raise your heart rate, make you slightly short of breath and get you sweating lightly – for thirty minutes three times a week may help reduce the number of painkillers you need to manage attacks. Aim for this amount of exercise as a good start and build it up, following your doctor's advice, if your migraine allows.

Yoga and tai chi

Yoga is a slower, mindful form of exercise that has been shown to help mood, control stress and improve depression and anxiety. A couple of studies from India have looked at whether yoga can help reduce migraine attacks too.[11]

Researchers have found that yoga's slow movements, and even the static, isometric muscle poses, combined with a clear mental focus on the activity are a beneficial addition to usual migraine care. Deep-breathing exercises in yoga, called **pranayama**, may also be helpful. This may be because deep breathing can stimulate the vagus nerve, which carries signals back and forth from the brain to the heart, lungs and gut. This nerve is part of the parasympathetic nervous system, sometimes called the 'rest and digest' system because it slows the heart and breathing rate while your gut moves food along during digestion.

If yoga interests you, it's probably wisest to find a class and talk to the instructor about your migraine before starting to practise. I would avoid dynamic yoga or hot yoga, to start with. Be careful with any poses or exercises that put strain on the neck. You may need to avoid or gradually build up to inverted postures and headstands. Practising what you have learned in class in your own time is important. Our brains take time to respond to these new techniques, and making them a regular habit will help reduce change in your routine.

Tai chi is a traditional Chinese exercise that has been practised for hundreds of years. Similar to yoga, its aim is to improve health, coordination and relaxation by going through flowing movements while maintaining mental focus. Tai chi has been shown to help with balance to prevent falls, mental health, stress relief and immune function. A study on tension-type headache found it to be generally helpful.[12] Another study, from Hong Kong, found that practising tai chi for one hour a day, five days a week for twelve weeks reduced the number of migraine days experienced each month significantly.[13]

Rebecca's story

Rebecca had had some success in controlling her episodic migraine attacks with various medications and daily swimming. But changes to her job and workplace meant she wouldn't be able to go swimming for a while. We talked through options to replace her swimming routine and she decided to try a weekly yoga class.

She made a commitment to practise regularly at home, aiming for half an hour most evenings. She found the calm of doing the stretches, postures and, in particular, the rhythmic breathing exercises really helped settle her brain at the end of a busy day. When we met again, she pulled out her migraine diary and showed me how she now needed fewer painkillers and was sleeping better too.

Taking exercise for your migraine doesn't require a big aerobic workout. In fact regular, gentle exercise like yoga can be helpful too and a good start.

Cold and heat

I sometimes ask patients in my clinic: When you have a migraine, which do you prefer – cold or heat? The range of answers I get is another strong confirmation of how much migraine varies from person to person and from attack to attack. Some of my patients tell me that using wrapped ice packs gives them relief, whereas others always reach for the warmth of a hot-water bottle. Some like both – heat on the shoulders and neck, a cold flannel on the forehead. Warmth on the back of the neck and shoulders may help to relax tense muscles.

In general, most people with migraine seem to find cold more helpful. The use of cold therapy for headaches has been described for more than 150 years. Today, cold can be applied quickly and efficiently with gels or freezable packs. One study looked at placing frozen neck-wraps over the carotid arteries at each side of the front of the neck where the strong pulse is felt, and 77 per cent of participants said this helped the pain and reduced the number of painkillers they had to take.[14]

If cold seems to work better for you, but gels and freezable packs aren't making much of a dent, then a soft hood-like product called Migra-Cap might be worth a try.[15] Wearing this freezable cap cools the front of the head, temples and back of the scalp all at the same time, delivering about forty-five minutes of relief. However, it also covers both eyes, so it's not something to wear out and about, but in the comfort of your home.

Menthol gel-sticks or pads, such as 4head or Kool'n'soothe, are more portable. Try them on the forehead when an attack starts or place them on painful neck muscles. It's worth noting that while some of my patients have found these helpful, those with heightened smell sensitivity say the menthol odour can be irritating, making an attack worse.

Some people find swimming in cold water – particularly 'wild swimming' outdoors – to be helpful in reducing their migraine headaches, and this approach has recently gained attention in the media.[16] The theory is that the combination of the shock of the cold water, the endorphin release that comes from the shock and the exercise, and the soothing effect of being out in nature reduces the experience of pain. There are many cold sensors in the skin, particularly around the mouth and nose, and immersing these areas in cold water may be stimulating the vagus nerve and activating the para-sympathetic nervous system, which settles us into 'rest and digest' mode. Being in spaces with lots of green vegetation and blue expanses of water is known to improve well-being too. Studies are needed to establish if it is immersing the face in cold water, exercising in cold conditions or the 'green-blue therapy' that is the most important factor.

It is, of course, essential to be safe. Sudden cold shock from immersion can trigger gasping, rapid breathing and even heart irregularities.[17] Check with your doctor if you have any doubts about your fitness to do cold-water swimming.

Your posture

Look around at other people, or ask someone to take a picture of you from one side as you stand upright. What you may notice is that many of us tend to have a posture where our head pokes forward from our neck, and our shoulders are rounded forward and sloping.

This head-forward posture is a result of a lot of time spent doing activities just in front of us – for example, cooking, writing or spending time on a computer or phone. Even talking to friends and family, we lean in. The head is heavy and so neck muscles have to hang on tight to maintain our head and neck position. Working muscles soon become tired and tense and may become painful. Improving this common posture may help to reduce the pain signals from the neck into the migraine-triggering centre of the brain. Researchers have found that there is an increased occurrence of musculoskeletal dysfunctions in people with migraine.

You can check your posture by standing with your back to a wall – how far away is the back of your head from the wall? Now make it touch the wall without tilting your chin up. For support, the head should be right above the cervical spine, and this allows the neck muscles to relax and soften. Notice also the position of your palms as you stand. If they face backwards, you are probably rounding your shoulders forward too much. Simply by turning both arms outwards from the shoulder, so that the palms face more towards the front, you will begin to get the feeling of a healthier, more upright posture.

Neck pain is a common symptom of migraine, reported by up to 76 per cent of people. One study found that people with migraine have increased neck-muscle stiffness.[18] Nerve fibres from the upper part of the spine, where your head and neck come together, join to form the **trigeminocervical complex** in the brain, an area involved in generating headache in migraine. I have often wondered whether exercises involving a lot of flexing or moving around the top of the spine might be more likely to trigger attacks. Boxing, weightlifting, breaststroke when swimming and anything that could give a form of whiplash movement, with sudden acceleration and then rapid stopping, might potentially send signals to irritate this area. Some of my patients report having an attack after certain gym exercises that target the neck and shoulders. After doing an endurance exercise where tension was maintained in the neck muscles against some resistance, 42 per cent of people in one study reported developing headache.[19]

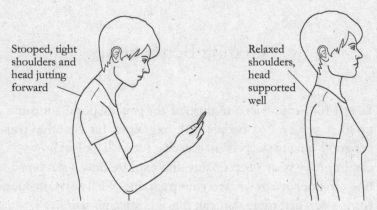

Stooped, tight shoulders and head jutting forward

Relaxed shoulders, head supported well

How most of us sit and stand (left), versus the hallmarks of good posture (right) – the spine and neck nice and long, the shoulders down and slightly back, with the head resting right above the spine, and the chin tucked down slightly

Once you have become more aware of your typical posture, there are many useful videos showing good posture on YouTube, which can help you learn how to foster a healthier relationship between your head, neck and shoulders. It's a good idea to see a physiotherapist or osteopath to help you strengthen the correct muscles too. New postures may feel odd at first, but exercises or classes like Pilates, which are designed to work on posture, can help you prevent the stooping posture and stiff neck that often arrive with increasing age. One study showed that Pilates exercises helped improve the head-forward posture and neck movement and also reduced neck and shoulder pain.[20] There are no studies looking at Pilates specifically for managing migraine at the time of writing. Discuss the options available in your area with your doctor or headache specialist.

5. Getting Better Sleep

Sleep problems affect one-third of the general population and up to 50 per cent of people with migraine.[1] It's vital that you get good-quality sleep. So in this chapter we'll look at how you can improve your sleep quality and explore how a sleep routine can improve or worsen your migraine. We'll also consider some sleep disorders that can make headaches worse.

Migraine and sleep

People with migraine probably need slightly more sleep than others. Fragmented or short nights of sleep can lead to tiredness, which may contribute to starting an attack,[2] and sleep quality is poorest in those with frequent or chronic migraine. People with migraine may frequently have trouble getting to sleep, have bad dreams or wake in the night or early morning. Pain can wake them too. Insomnia, restless legs syndrome (RLS), snoring and teeth-grinding (bruxism) are also common.

Some people find going to sleep relieves their migraine, but many others report that having a lie-in, and extending sleep beyond their usual hours, is a powerful migraine trigger. The resulting attack may build up over a few days. A number of my patients realize, like a light-bulb moment, that this explains their Monday-morning headaches: that luxurious, lazy Saturday-morning sleep was the tipping point. Travelling by air often upsets sleep routine and quality – one reason many people get attacks in the first days of their holiday.

Good-quality sleep and a regular bedtime routine are especially important for the brain of a person with migraine, but sleep experts explain it is a myth that adults all need eight hours of sleep.[3] Individuals vary, with some needing nine hours and others being fine after only six. You are sleeping enough if you're not tired the next day, assuming that no other medical conditions make you feel fatigued.

Normal sleep phases are well understood. Sleep is divided into rapid eye movement (REM) and non-REM sleep. These phases alter the depth of your sleep throughout the night and occur in ninety-minute cycles. Many people wear electronic wrist devices like the Fitbit to count steps, to remind them to move or even to check their heartbeat rhythms. Don't be tempted to use them to track your sleep, though. Although they promise a wealth of data about your sleep, the information is unreliable and may cause sleep anxiety. Sleep experts advise that you take off your Fitbit at bedtime.

Migraine pain and sleep are intimately interconnected in the brain. When normal sleep is disrupted and you are sleep-deprived, the brain's pain centres can become irritated and can heighten your awareness of pain. Conversely, chronic pain affecting nerve cells (neurons) in the brain can disturb your sleep cycle. The hypothalamus – one of the brain structures known to be involved in generating attacks – is important in sleep regulation too. Neurons in the hypothalamus produce a neurochemical called orexin, which plays a role in both controlling sleep/wake cycles and modulating pain. Low levels of the hormone melatonin, produced by the pineal gland in the brain and also involved in daily sleep/wake cycles, have been associated with chronic migraine.[4]

So it's not surprising that insomnia and migraine have a bi-directional relationship, with one affecting the other. **Insomnia**, the inability to fall or stay asleep at night, is the most common sleep disorder. People with insomnia may also have depression or anxiety, with these sometimes causing their sleep disorder and sometimes being caused by it.[5] Either way, the gold-standard treatment is **cognitive behavioural therapy for insomnia** (CBTi). This technique, which is often taught by a psychologist, can also be explored through online courses, apps or books.

The first strategy is to 'anchor your day'. Fix a waking-up time and stick to it every day, even at weekends. Your sleep 'fuel', a hormone called adenosine, builds up during the day until it's high enough to make you feel sleepy. That's the best time to go to bed – just as you start to feel drowsy. Using your bed as a workplace or amusement centre trains your brain to associate being in bed with being active.

Relaxation techniques and other strategies may also be covered in a CBTi course. Although it may take a few weeks to settle into healthier, better-quality sleep, be patient and practise until you form new habits. Many people have found these techniques really improve their sleep.

> <u>**Tips for improving sleep**</u>
> * **Work out how many hours of sleep you need and stick to it. Beware the lie-in.**
> * **Your sleep/wake cycle is helped by being out in daylight. This sets your body clock.**

- Exercise can help you sleep, but not just before bedtime.
- Wind down an hour before bedtime and dim the lights. Don't train your brain to be alert in bed by watching TV, checking your phone or playing games there.
- Avoid stimulants. Keep caffeine for the mornings or avoid it altogether. Don't smoke – nicotine is a stimulant too. Limit or avoid alcohol, as this can disrupt sleep cycles.
- Where possible, keep your bedroom for getting dressed and undressed, sleep and intimacy – leave electronic devices in another room.

Henry's story

Henry is managing director of his company. After waking at 6.30 a.m., he grabs a coffee on his drive to the office, the first of three (or five) he has each day. He says they fuel him. He's typically at his computer or on the phone for hours at a stretch. By the time the weekend rolls around, he's exhausted. He really looks forward to winding down on Friday evening with some wine and then relaxing on Saturday – no alarm clock going off at 6.30. But all too often his weekend will be spoiled by a migraine attack coming on later in the day.

We discussed changes he could try to avoid these regular 'let-down' headaches. These included limiting his coffee intake to one or two cups before lunch. He decided to walk around the block every lunchtime for some fresh air and exercise. He changed his sleep routine so that he was waking at a similar time every day, which took a bit of adjustment. But as his reward, his migraine attacks became less frequent and he flagged less at work.

Taking a holistic approach to improving your sleep is essential. As you adjust to a more regular sleep routine, keep an eye out for stimulants that might disrupt your sleep – not just caffeine, but also nicotine, alcohol and stress (good and bad).

Other sleep disorders

There are many sleep disorders beyond insomnia, including narcolepsy (daytime sleepiness and sleep attacks), shift-work sleep disorder and jet lag. For people with migraine, some other conditions affecting sleep are worth closer discussion.

- **Obstructive sleep apnoea:** Do you snore loudly or ever wake with a start, gasping for air? Heavy snorers may have a condition called obstructive sleep apnoea (OSA).

  Snoring occurs when the back of the nose and throat relax and fall back while a person goes into deep sleep. In OSA their airway gets partially, then fully, blocked, and breathing gets louder and noisier and then pauses. Carbon dioxide builds up in the blood, eventually triggering a strong urge to breathe – waking them with a gasp and a jolt. This cycle may repeat many times during the night. Sometimes the person only partially wakes and doesn't realize what has happened. The following day they feel drained.

People with OSA may not even know they snore, let alone stop breathing. The description often comes from a sleeping partner, who complains they 'wake with a snort' or 'need a nudge to start breathing again'. The condition is more common as people get older and in men, overweight people and those with a large collar size, but it can also occur in women and even children, especially those with large tonsils and adenoids. People with OSA often wake with a bad morning headache.[6] In many people who get these headaches, migrainous features occur too.[7]

If you or your sleeping partner suspects you may have OSA, take the online STOP-Bang Questionnaire (stopbang.ca/osa/screening.php). If you score highly on this, ask your family doctor to refer you for a sleep study to see if you need treatment. This study may be done at home using equipment to measure your breathing patterns and oxygen levels while you sleep. In some cases a more detailed sleep study is done in hospital.

OSA can also lead to high blood pressure and increased risk of heart problems if it is not sorted out. So please take snoring seriously.

- **Restless legs syndrome**: Migraine is linked with another condition that can impact sleep – restless legs syndrome (RLS), also known as Willis–Ekbom disease. This is the almost indescribable and unpleasant feeling of needing to move the legs, which is only relieved when the legs are actually moved. It usually starts in the evening and can occur repeatedly and into the night, greatly impacting on sleep quality. RLS is linked to iron deficiency, so ask your doctor about getting blood tests to check this, if you think you may have it.

- **Hypnic headache**: This is a rare type of headache that occurs exclusively during sleep.[8] A dull, featureless headache that comes on in the night and wakes the person from sleep, it affects mainly women in midlife or older. Often sufferers have a history of migraine. Curiously, having caffeine just before sleeping seems to help hypnic headache.[9]

Many sleep problems are worse with stress. The mind gets busy thinking about things and this disrupts your rest. In the next chapter we'll be looking at techniques for managing this.

6. Managing Your Mental Health

Most people with migraine have been told, 'It's probably because you're stressed.' I've certainly had stress proposed as the cause of my attacks. I dislike this phrase, which seems to blame the sufferer, implying they aren't coping, or they should 'chill out', and all will be well. Yet stress reduction has a central place in many successful migraine-management plans.

It's also important to acknowledge and treat mental-health conditions. One study found that mild to moderate depressive symptoms were present in 47 per cent of people with migraine.[1] The relationship between migraine and mental health is complicated but treatable.

In this chapter we look at physical and emotional factors that may put stress on our brains and explore possible strategies for reducing this. We also consider how mental-health conditions, especially anxiety and depression, commonly coexist with migraine, and what can help. Family life can be affected too.

What is 'stress' to a migraine brain?

As mentioned in Chapter 2, the brain of a person with migraine is genetically programmed to react abnormally to psychological and physiological changes, being hyper-excitable even between attacks. Over time, prolonged stress can increase migraine frequency and ultimately move you from having episodic migraine attacks to chronic migraine.

Light, visual patterns, smells and sounds are **physical stressors** that can irritate the migraine brain. Many patients of mine have reduced light-glare impact by turning down the brightness on computer screens, downloading software to reduce screen glare, using 'dark mode' on phones or wearing tinted glasses, such as MigraLens, TheraSpecs or Avulux. A wide-brimmed hat outside and a pair of sunglasses may reduce glare from the sun. Fluorescent lights may need to be switched off or shielded and replaced by desk lamps.

Stripes and high-contrast patterns like checks have been shown to irritate some people. One five-year-old patient asked his mum to move his sister's school dress, hanging on the back of the door, because he could not look at the chequered gingham fabric without feeling very uncomfortable and migrainous.

Avoiding strong smells may be relatively easy to do at home, but harder when you're at work or out and about, where exposure to perfume fragrances, food odours and diesel fumes will be trickier to control. Headphones or earplugs can help reduce stress from external noises. Blaring music should be turned down, where possible.

Reducing these physical stressors can make your brain feel more comfortable, reduce the chance of an attack starting and help one to settle quickly.

People sometimes refer to themselves as 'stressed out', and **emotional stressors** are a ubiquitous feature of modern life. Good stress is exciting or challenging; bad stress leads to worry or frustration.

Stress affects the body through chemical mediators, including the hormones adrenaline and glucocorticosteroid, produced by the adrenal glands. Release of these hormones gives the typical physical reactions and feelings that we associate with stress: a dry mouth, rapid heart rate, stomach churning and feelings of anxiety or panic. These can be helpful, enabling us to flee or take protective action if danger is near and real, or unhelpful if the response is prolonged or out of proportion to the actual threat.

When we're 'stressed out', prolonged bad stress can overwhelm our body's coping mechanisms, gradually leading to illness.

Stress hormones: good news, bad news

Good news, initially . . .

* Concentration and memory are enhanced.
* New strategies to help us feel safe can be learned.
* Food-seeking behaviour gives us energy sources and strength.
* Immune defence mechanisms are activated.

Bad news, if stress is prolonged . . .

* Nerve cells and memory processing may be weakened or damaged.
* Comfort-eating can lead to insulin resistance, which leads to obesity and increases the risk of heart disease and other conditions.
* Sleep quality worsens.
* The immune system can be suppressed, increasing the risk of becoming unwell from bacterial and viral infections.
* Migraine may worsen and become chronic.

Stress, both good and bad, is one of the most commonly cited triggers for worsening migraine. But because a combination of triggers starts an attack, blaming stress alone is not helpful.

Migraine is a fluctuating, lifelong condition, and stressful life events – changing jobs, moving house, experiencing financial difficulties or family strife – often increase the frequency of attacks.

The wear and tear of chronic stress on our bodies and brains can provoke migraine and mood disorders like depression and anxiety. By understanding this, we can begin to see what might help. We can't always stop emotional stressors from being in our lives. Our work/life balance and unpredictable major life events regularly throw us into stressful situations. But we can pay attention to how we react to stressors, reducing their impact.

Habitual responses are hard to change. It may take time to find stress-reduction techniques that suit you and fit into your life. Aim to be patient, and persevere in your efforts to find calm.

Self-management

There are a number of stress-reduction techniques that can be explored at home.

- **Breath awareness**: Simple relaxation techniques can work as instant stress-relievers. We tend to breathe too fast, taking rapid breaths into the upper part of the chest, tightening our neck and shoulder muscles, when anxious or tense. Our calming, parasympathetic nervous system is activated when we breathe out slowly. Slowing breathing down, especially as we exhale, and using our abdominal muscles to breathe, helps calm us and reduces adrenaline. Many YouTube videos, apps, books and podcasts will teach you how to do this. A number are guided by a gentle voice and specifically aim to help you relax into sleep. Some people like the soothing sounds of rainfall or whale music. I prefer peace and quiet during relaxation breathing exercises. Find one you like and start to practise.

- **Mindfulness and meditation**: There are three core components to meditation: attention control, emotional regulation and self-awareness. Studies of people with migraine using mindfulness and other types of meditation have shown that these may help reduce headache intensity.[2] Research confirms that, with regular practice, the activating areas of the brain settle, sleep quality improves and pain reduces.

One popular programme, which can be learned through books and online or in-person courses, is **mindfulness-based stress reduction** (MBSR). This trains you to:

- Concentrate fully on the present moment.
- Avoid judging yourself.
- Be aware of your breath.

During mindfulness meditation, our minds often chatter at us. Some patients complain that they are useless at it and too easily distracted. This experience is normal. If you experience this when attempting mindfulness, you are not failing. The idea is to *notice* that your thoughts have wandered, before returning to the gentle observation of your body or your breaths. An inner stillness gradually results, with greater awareness of the present moment in whatever you're doing. Many people find benefit simply from stopping to do a meditation every day for ten to forty minutes. MBSR can be practised while eating or walking too.

Researchers have found that spiritual meditation seems to improve pain tolerance too.[3] Generally, meditation practised regularly seems to give positive physical and psychological effects.

To get into the habit of being mindful, I sometimes suggest to my overly busy, stressed-out patients that they take a fifteen-minute holiday every day – no travelling necessary!

- **Mindfulness-based cognitive therapy (MBCT)**: Our thoughts affect our feelings and how we behave. MBCT focuses more on the way we perceive our migraine and how this influences our behaviour.

  Sometimes the way we think about our migraine can be unhelpful. An example is 'catastrophizing', where you think: 'I'm never going to get rid of my migraine. I'll always be suffering.' A more helpful self-message might be, 'My migraine is bad at the moment, but hopefully it will ease soon. Research is happening that might help me in the future. I know migraine can come and go over time too.' Changing your perception of pain might help you reduce its impact on your daily life.

Your family doctor can advise you about getting MBCT sessions, which are usually led by a psychologist. Useful self-help resources like the Pain Toolkit (paintoolkit.org) or the Pain Management Plan (pain-management-plan.co.uk) are also well worth trying.

These techniques can help teach you to be kind to yourself, to judge yourself less harshly and to feel less guilty about having a chronic condition. We are often far more critical of ourselves than of others, so remember to practise self-compassion.

- **Expressive writing**: Sometimes called 'therapeutic journaling', expressive writing has been shown to be helpful with chronic pain, mental-health issues and migraine.[4] Unexpected life events, trauma and stress can lead to repetitive worrying thoughts and dwelling on past events. Privately exploring thoughts, feelings and past events through writing can help reduce ruminating over painful occurrences. Voicing your distress on paper can also sometimes help you share difficult emotions with others, but this is not the primary aim. If you feel the stress around a particular event in your life has added to your migraine frequency or severity, you may find this technique helpful.

  Gratitude journaling, keeping a daily note of several things you are thankful for – be they large or small – can improve positivity, reduce stress and improve sleep too.[5]

  <u>**Expressive-writing exercise**</u>
  Sit for fifteen to twenty minutes each day for four consecutive days. Use pen and paper, rather

than a computer. Write freely about an important issue for you. Don't stop writing, or worry about spelling or punctuation. Focus on what is particularly on your mind. Release difficult emotions in your writing. If it comes naturally, write about possible solutions. Don't reread what you have written or share it with anyone. Instead, after you're done writing, shred the paper or throw it away securely.

- **Hypnotherapy**: This is the therapeutic use of hypnosis to induce a state of deep relaxation. Under hypnosis the brain becomes more open to suggestion, and this has been used to help change unhelpful thought patterns and reduce anxiety. Unfortunately the spectacle of volunteers being hypnotized onstage has scared off a lot of people. But don't worry – hypnosis can't make you lose control over your mind; no one can make you do something you don't want to while you're hypnotized. The British Society of Clinical Hypnosis (bsch.org.uk), the American Society of Clinical Hypnosis (asch.net) and other national bodies have lists of registered, vetted clinical hypnotherapists. A number of studies have shown that hypnotherapy can help migraine.[6]
- **Exercise**: Don't forget, exercise is one of the best ways to beat stress. A walk in the morning helps to keep your body clock (circadian rhythm) on track. In addition to the health benefits for migraine that we saw in Chapter 4, researchers have found that physical activity in green

spaces like parks or woods is more beneficial for improving psychological and emotional well-being than exercising indoors, even in winter.[7] So dress for the weather and get moving outside if you can.

Amina's story

Tearfully, Amina told me how she hated her migraine attacks. She worried constantly about getting one, especially around family events. Her large family loved to celebrate special days together and she was often enlisted as the organizer – a role she'd once relished. But as a party drew closer, she'd get anxious that she would have an attack and let everyone down. She was sure this dread was now causing her to have attacks more readily.

She didn't want to give up being involved in family events, so we discussed a rescue treatment plan. She referred herself for some cognitive behavioural therapy (CBT) and started meditating for fifteen minutes a day, using an app she liked. The CBT helped her to reframe her thoughts and plan how she would manage if she did have an attack on a party day. The meditation app introduced her to some simple visualization exercises to try when she felt her anxiety rising. Together, they greatly reduced her anticipatory anxiety. Her attacks began to have less impact on her, and on her relationships with her family.

Like a migraine attack, stress can snowball. Finding techniques that help you be more aware of stress and manage it will help you quash stress before it gets a chance to build up and take its toll.

Mental-health conditions and migraine

Anxiety and mood disorders are very common in people with migraine. They can influence attack severity and treatment response, and can have a long-term impact on people's lives. If not recognized and treated properly, they can lead to chronic migraine and can worsen the disability associated with frequent and severe attacks.

Anxiety occurs up to five times more frequently in people with migraine than in those without.[8] This may be felt as generalized anxiety, obsessional compulsive disorder (OCD) or panic disorder. I often hear my patients describe 'anticipatory anxiety' – intense worry in advance of an event, like a wedding or an important work presentation, that an attack will ruin the day. This can contribute to an attack starting, reinforcing and amplifying their anxiety in future. When a personalized migraine treatment plan works to improve control of anxiety as well as migraine in people experiencing both, life becomes easier.

Depression is 2.5 times more likely to occur in a person with migraine, and more people with depression get migraine than the general population.[9] The association is even higher in people with chronic migraine or migraine with aura. There seem to be some common processes in the brain that link these conditions. Some medications that doctors prescribe for depression are also used for migraine. If you have both, this might guide your decision about which medication to try first.

Bipolar disorder and migraine are also associated. There is probably a genetic link but the reason is not yet fully understood. People with migraine have been found to be three times more likely to have bipolar disorder, and one-third of people with bipolar also suffer from migraine.[10]

Adverse childhood experiences (ACEs) and **abuse** are frequently associated with migraine. Child abuse – whether physical, emotional, sexual or neglect – increases the risk of developing migraine,[11] as does any major stressful life event. Again this may be due to the effect of the stress hormones adrenaline and glucocorticosteroid, and it appears it is not the trauma alone but also the development of **post-traumatic stress disorder (PTSD)** that is key. PTSD heightens the effect of trauma by increasing the reactivity and sensitivity of pain pathways in the brain. Often people with PTSD take more painkilling medication as a result. It may be that the brain processes leading to migraine make PTSD more likely to occur after traumatic events.

All these mental-health conditions are treatable. Medications or interventions such as counselling, CBT, mindfulness meditation and exercise may help. If you feel you may have any of the above conditions in addition to migraine, then it's really important to recognize this and seek help. Ask your family doctor about recommended therapists and treatment options that you can get in your area. Finding the right help for you as an individual can take a while, but it will be worth it in the long term.

The impact on families

Migraine, especially chronic migraine, ripples out to affect more people than just the sufferer. It impacts relationships and family life too. The MAZE survey found that people with migraine were less able to do normal household tasks, sometimes only just struggling through by doing them slowly.[12] They miss more days of family, social or leisure activities than work/school days.

Interacting with children or partners can be disrupted. Planned family activities may have to be cancelled, or may go ahead without the person with migraine. I remember clearly lying in bed on the first day of a family holiday while everyone else went out to explore. There may be a financial impact on the household, if migraine impacts a person's ability to work or progress in their career.

The Impact of Migraine on Partners and Adolescent Children (IMPAC) Scale was developed to measure this and see how help can be better provided.[13] If you feel your migraine is affecting your family, for example, because your headaches kick off arguments or cause plans to be cancelled, you may want to fill out the IMPAC Scale and bring it with you when you meet your doctor or headache specialist. It can be a good starting point for a conversation about strategies and support to help lighten the burden on both you and your family.

There are also support programmes for people with migraine, including those listed in the Further Reading and

Resources (see page 211). One highly effective programme, the Migraine Youth Camp, was set up for teenagers and their families in the US to help them learn about migraine and reduce their feelings of isolation.[14] Ask your doctor or headache specialist if a local support group offers something similar. New initiatives are being launched each year.

7. Rescue Plans for Acute Attacks

If you have a migraine brain, you may try to control every-thing you can – what you eat, how you exercise, when you sleep and how you respond to stress – but an attack may still come. When the aura flickers, the nausea starts or the head-ache begins to pound, what do you reach for?

It's now time to look at the main choices for treating your migraine attacks. Finding a rescue plan that works well for your particular attacks might take a while, as every brain responds differently to medications and therapies. What suits your friend or family member may not work for you. And some medications can make things worse. This is important to take in. It's a reason why you should never take someone else's medication – no matter how desperate you are or how well-meaning they may be in offering it to you.

We'll also take a closer look at medication-overuse head-ache, a problem that often brings new patients to my clinic at the National Migraine Centre. In many cases they have not been given clear advice about how many painkillers is too many. Confused, they sometimes delay their medication until too late, when they are less likely to get relief.

For medication to work, it must reach the right place, at the right time and at the right dose.

The right place

A migraine attack needs to be treated with the best painkiller for you, but this also needs to reach the best place in your gut to be rapidly absorbed. As we saw in Chapter 2, in migraine the brain slows down muscle activity in the gut to a dysfunctional level, a condition called **gastric stasis**, or gastroparesis. This happens because of the migraine's influence on the vagus nerve, which runs from the brain to the heart, lungs and gut. In people with migraine, gastric stasis occurs both during and *between* attacks. This dysfunction of the gut is an important feature of migraine to understand if you want to treat your attacks with medication.

The vagus nerve works on smooth muscles in the gut wall to alter how quickly food and medication move through your stomach. In gastric stasis, it simply takes much longer to empty the stomach. The result is that about 30 per cent of people with migraine report vomiting, and around 70 per cent suffer nausea during an attack.[1] Symptoms range from mild queasiness or bloating through to violent, repeated vomiting attacks lasting a few days. Of course a significant consequence is that any medications that you have swallowed to reduce your pain get held up in your stomach, and this is not where they are optimally absorbed into the bloodstream. They need to move on to the small intestine. The upshot: your migraine grows in severity and it feels as if those drugs don't work.

To help push the medication into the right place, you can ask your doctor or headache specialist to prescribe **anti-emetics**, drugs that stop nausea and vomiting even if you don't experience these symptoms. These are so helpful to people with migraine and yet, surprisingly, I find my patients have often not been offered them by their family doctor. The most helpful anti-emetics for migraine are 'prokinetic', which means they work by strengthening the contractions of the muscles in the stomach wall to push the contents along in the right direction. Other anti-emetics work indirectly in the brain by suppressing the feeling of nausea. This may be helpful, enabling you to eat and drink, but they won't speed up the absorption of painkillers.

Anti-emetics can be taken as tablets, sometimes in a dissolvable form that is placed between the gum and the inner cheek, by suppository or by injection.

The right time

You should take your migraine medication as soon as you are aware that an attack is coming on. The longer you leave it, the more momentum the migraine gathers and the more pain and symptoms you will feel. Returning to my snowball analogy from Chapter 2, if you want to stop a big snowball from bowling you over, you need to squash it as it starts to roll, rather than waiting until it has gathered momentum and is heading down the mountainside right towards you! Taking medication early reduces the chances of an attack wiping you out for a day or two.

The trouble with this strategy is that it isn't always that easy to tell if you have a bad migraine coming or a milder one that will ease off by itself. Some of my patients struggle with this, as they are aware they should not use any painkillers too frequently, to reduce the risk of developing medication-overuse headaches. However, many of the medications prescribed for migraine can safely be repeated within twenty-four hours if you have attacks that tend to roll on from one day to another. Rechecking whether your migraine is developing or dissipating, an hour after you take simple painkillers, can help you decide if you need a stronger triptan medication (see page 95) to get rid of it.

Only use the doses recommended by the doctor, nurse or pharmacist who is advising you about your migraine. Don't be tempted to break tablets in half to eke them out, either. That's not a good idea – half the dose for two days is less likely to be an effective rescue and increases your risk of developing medication-overuse headache.

The right dose

The dose you take will depend on the particular medication you are using, and it would not be right to give specific doses of drugs here. You need to discuss the right dose for you with your doctor or headache specialist.

The general rule is that you need the maximum power of the drug as close to the start of the migraine as possible. You need to hit the symptoms hard. At the same time, be aware that it's possible to overdose on drugs, particularly painkillers. So you need to check with your doctor or headache specialist about a safe 'starter' dose for each medication that you try, and note how long you need to wait before repeating the dose.

Can an over-the-counter painkiller be enough?

The availability of medicines for migraine varies around the world. In some places, strict rules govern the supply of certain painkillers used for migraine. In other countries you may be able to buy the same drugs from a local pharmacy. In most countries aspirin (acetylsalicylic acid), paracetamol (acetaminophen) and ibuprofen are easily available to buy.

Aspirin seems to be particularly helpful for migraine, especially for the aura phase. On the whole, non-steroidal anti-inflammatory drugs (NSAIDs) like ibuprofen are more effective than paracetamol. However, one review found that the effect of paracetamol was enhanced if the person also took the anti-emetic metoclopramide to treat their gastric stasis.[2] Which one you choose will, of course, need to be decided with regard also to other medications, allergies or medical conditions you have.

The formulation in which you take these can affect how they work. Simple tablets have to dissolve in your gut, and this takes time – with or without gastric stasis. To speed things up, many of these drugs are also available in soluble or liquid form. Taking effervescent tablets that fizz, or adding a tablet that dissolves to a fizzy drink, will not only speed up the dissolving process but also allows the active ingredients to be spread over a larger surface area in your gut, helping to get them into your bloodstream all the sooner.

Colas containing sugar and caffeine may be useful, because the sugar ensures the brain has enough glucose fuel, and the caffeine can boost the pain-relieving effect of the medication. I have had patients tell me that having a strong coffee with their painkillers really does the trick. Many over-the-counter painkillers contain caffeine for this co-analgesic effect.

If you have chosen to cut caffeine out of your diet as a possible trigger, be sure to read the small print on the labels for over-the-counter painkillers.

Triptans

There are also several medications prescribed specifically for migraine called **triptans**.

The first triptan developed was sumatriptan, and this medication is still used widely today, three decades after it was first approved for use. It can be taken as a tablet, a nasal spray or an injection. Since then, six other triptans have been licensed: naratriptan, zolmitriptan, rizatriptan, almotriptan, eletriptan and frovatriptan. The table overleaf outlines some of their properties and formulations.

As both a doctor and a person with migraine, I have found that not all triptans work equally well for everybody. One may work very well for me, where another isn't effective. It's impossible to look at a person and know which triptan will work for them. If you try one and it doesn't suit you, it's worth working through others to see if another triptan can be part of your rescue plan.

Your triptan choice might also vary according to the situation you're in when an attack starts. If you're about to have a job interview or take an exam, you might need a fast-acting nasal spray or melt tablet (oro-dispersible). If you know you're about to have a menstrual period, and that means you can expect a long attack lasting three days or more, a longer-acting triptan like naratriptan or frovatriptan might be more useful.

Triptan	Formulations available	Duration of action
Sumatriptan	Tablet, nasal spray, injection	Short
Almotriptan	Tablet	Short
Eletriptan	Tablet	Short
Rizatriptan	Tablet, oro-dispersible (melt)	Short
Zolmitriptan	Tablet, oro-dispersible (melt), nasal spray	Short
Naratriptan	Tablet	Medium
Frovatriptan	Tablet	Long

The triptans and their properties[3]

Triptans can interact with some other medications and are not advised in people with heart conditions. They are not licensed for use in those aged sixty-five or older.

The price of triptans varies widely and, certainly in the UK, some doctors are constrained by local prescribing budgets as to which triptans they might be able to offer. Talk with your doctor or headache specialist about your options and needs and make the decision together.

Current guidelines in the UK and elsewhere suggest that people take an anti-emetic, a painkiller and a triptan together, when a moderate to severe migraine is starting.[4] You need to know your own pattern of migraine and decide at the beginning of each attack whether you take the anti-emetic and a simple painkiller, or whether you take all three at once.

Judging the severity of a migraine at the start of an attack can be hard, but doing so may help you avoid overusing medication, which can become a problem in itself. If you have decided to keep a triptan in reserve, don't wait too long before adding it, if you feel your symptoms mounting. I suggest waiting just forty-five minutes to see if the simple painkillers have worked. If they haven't, don't miss the boat – take the triptan. And if you wake up with a migraine, take all three at the same time, as the migraine already has you in its grip.

Milly's story

Milly was getting occasional migraine with aura. She felt queasy during attacks. She was confused about painkillers. She knew taking too many could be a problem, so she waited until her headache was really bad before taking paracetamol. It never worked. Her doctor had suggested a triptan, but it always made her sleepy, which meant she couldn't take it while she was at work or looking after her children.

We discussed tackling her migraine attacks as quickly as possible with the right medication, in the right place, at the right time. I added a medication to reduce her nausea and help absorption of the painkillers. She found that what often worked was taking her anti-nausea pill along with soluble aspirin dissolved in Coca-Cola as soon as her aura started. If her headache grew despite this, forty-five minutes later she took a triptan – a different one from the pill that made her sleepy. This rescue plan enabled her to quickly stop her attacks before they snowballed.

It may take time to find the right combination of medications and timings. Keep trying.

Status migrainosus

Sometimes a migraine episode seems to linger longer than the usual attack. I've had patients in my clinic complain, 'This migraine has been around for a couple of weeks. I can't seem to get rid of it.' When a typical attack is severe and unremitting and lasts for more than seventy-two hours, it can be classified as **status migrainosus**. A prolonged severe attack like this often has a serious and significant impact on day-to-day activities, sleep and mood.

In these attacks, symptoms may fluctuate and ease for up to twelve hours following medication or sleep, but then they come back relentlessly. Sometimes medication overuse can lead to headaches like this, or they may mark a transition from episodic to chronic migraine.

To treat this, doctors may prescribe a regular dose of a non-steroidal anti-inflammatory medication like naproxen to be taken three times a day for a number of weeks. This may help but, if the headache continues to be resistant to the normal treatments you use at home, it may be necessary to have treatment in hospital by intravenous injection of stronger medication. Thankfully, this is rare.

Novel medications

The discovery of the integral role of the neurochemical calcitonin gene-related peptide (CGRP) in migraine attacks has led to the development of promising new lines of treatment, both for treating acute attacks and for preventing attacks from occurring.

There are two types of CGRP-based drugs for treating acute attacks: the so-called gepants and the ditans. Both are considered to be alternatives to triptans. They seem to be safer in people with cardiovascular risk factors, for whom triptans would not be advised.

The gepant group includes ubrogepant and rimegepant. These are **CGRP receptor antagonists**, which means they block or reduce the ability of CGRP to bind to cells, stopping activation of the pain pathway. Side-effects reported in trials include nausea. They are taken by mouth.

The ditan lasmiditan works on a similar receptor in the brain as triptans, but doesn't constrict blood vessels like triptans can do. Side-effects include dizziness and tingling (paraesthesia). It is taken by mouth.

These drugs were approved for use in the US in 2019 and 2020, with the expectation that they will be approved in other countries shortly. At the time of writing they were not yet available in the UK.

Alternatives to tablets

I have some patients who really dislike using rescue medications, or who can't take them because their body can't tolerate them or the medications aren't compatible with other medical conditions or medications. The good news is that there are other strategies that can help treat an acute migraine attack. Among these are **neuromodulation devices**, which work by influencing the brain pathways that lead to an attack.

One such device is called the Cefaly Dual. It is placed with a special adhesive pad on the centre of the forehead, between the eyes. Wearing it, you look a little like a character from *Star Trek*! There are buttons on the front, which you use to regulate electrical impulses generated by the machine. These impulses spread out over the supraorbital and supratrochlear nerves, which lie on each side of your face, above your eyebrows. This electrical stimulation stops your brain receiving strong signals from these nerves and may quiet your attack. For use as a rescue, you need to put it on near the onset and wear it for an hour. It is very safe, with virtually no side-effects, and has good results for some people. I've had a few patients in my clinic who find it soothing. Others dislike the buzzing feeling it generates, especially if they have a sensitive scalp. Cefaly Dual is not covered by all health services or insurance plans, so in most cases you will need to buy it yourself. It is a relatively expensive treatment option but, at the time of writing, the manufacturer offers a partial refund if it doesn't suit you.

Exploring neuromodulation therapies led to the development of the sTMS mini device, which uses magnetic rather than electric pulses to calm brain irritability in people with migraine. This device is held at the base of the skull at the back of the head. Several of my patients who have tried it say it can feel like a jolt inside the head, but this is not unpleasant. It's also safe and well tolerated. Unfortunately, the company that developed the device stopped manufacturing it in 2020. Given the early successful reports, some people with migraine are hopeful the technology might be used again in the future, so it might be worth keeping an eye out for it in case it becomes available once more.

A third neuromodulation device, the Nerivio, is not placed on the head but is instead wrapped around the upper arm.

Electrical impulses from this device travel along the nerves of the arm up to the brain. The specific frequency of the signals has been found to help diminish migraine pain. It has already been approved for use in the US and may be launched in the UK soon.

Nerve blocks are sometimes used to cut short a severe migraine attack by injection of a nerve-numbing local anaesthetic into the back of the scalp. The availability of a trained specialist during your attack is a practical, limiting factor, though.

Finally, don't forget the power of the simple physical interventions that we considered in Chapters 2 and 4, such as going into a dark room, or using cold or heat, to soothe your brain.

Medications to avoid

There is one class of medication that headache specialists actively discourage people from taking: opiates. This class of painkillers includes codeine, morphine, tramadol and codeine-based compound medications like co-codamol (a compound of codeine and paracetamol), Solpadeine and Migraleve. Opiates are addictive, sedative and poorly effective for migraine pain and they exacerbate gastric stasis. They are just not well suited for treating migraine.

Some patients searching for some way to ease a severe headache try codeine. Sometimes a doctor who is not a headache specialist may have prescribed it – for example, if you've gone to the emergency department. In many places, including the UK, codeine-containing medications are easily available to buy and some are specifically marketed as being for migraine. I strongly advise you not to be tempted. These types of medication can rapidly transform episodic migraine into chronic migraine. They are also more likely to provoke medication-overuse headache, which is even harder to treat.

If you did not realize this and have been taking codeine or other opiates frequently, talk to your doctor or headache specialist about coming off them slowly. The addictive nature of these drugs means that you can experience withdrawal symptoms if you reduce them too quickly.

Medication-overuse headache

Sensitivity to painkilling medication seems to be a particular characteristic of the brain of people with migraine. **Medication-overuse headache** (MOH) is a common secondary headache caused by taking painkillers on too many days each month. Any of the medications commonly used to treat pain can cause it.

When I see patients in my clinic, one clue that they may have developed MOH comes when I hear, 'My migraine attacks used to come occasionally, but now they come more and more frequently – my painkillers don't work any more' or 'The pain is there almost every day, but sometimes I get really bad days.' I have to stop myself from pulling a wry face when I hear, 'I have been taking codeine, but nothing works any more.'

The best way to avoid getting MOH is to know about it before you start treating your migraine with painkillers. Unfortunately all too often this information isn't given. Even where it has been, it can too easily be overlooked among instructions about timings and doses. You are not to blame if you have developed this troublesome condition. It's a by-product of trying to rescue yourself from the worst of your symptoms. And while prevention is best for avoiding medication-overuse headache, this condition can also be treated.

I find the simplest way to ensure you're not taking too much medication is to think in days, not doses. This switch in how you think is important – particularly in the way you handle taking your medication when you do. Don't break tablets in half to spread a dose out over a few days. The brain of a person with migraine is much more irritated by small, frequent doses over several days than by higher doses concentrated in one twenty-four-hour period. Certain medications are also much more likely to cause MOH than others. I suggest that my patients stick to these guidelines:

- Simple painkillers like aspirin, paracetamol, ibuprofen and naproxen: take these on a maximum of fourteen days per month.
- Triptans: take these on a maximum of eight days per month.
- Codeine and opiates: as these are the most likely to lead to MOH, avoid them altogether.

The days of effective treatment can be consecutive or spread out, so long as you don't exceed the total days per month.

If you've already developed MOH, treatment involves stopping the painkillers you have been taking. You'll probably need some guidance and support from a doctor, nurse or other headache specialist as you go through this detoxing process.

Sometimes the brain reacts to this loss of medication by becoming more irritable for a while, and it may feel as if the migraine is simply getting worse and worse for a couple of weeks. The clear days will begin to come eventually. Recovery from triptan overuse usually takes about four to six weeks. If you've been taking codeine it may take up to six months, and you may need to reduce it more slowly because of withdrawal symptoms. Tackling MOH can feel daunting, but do persevere. In my clinic I've had many patients who initially baulked at the thought of not taking painkillers for a few weeks, but have seen rewarding improvements in their migraine frequency and severity by following through.

If you've been having MOH, status migrainosus or high-frequency episodic attacks, it's time to look beyond your rescue plan to preventive medication and treatments.

8. Migraine Preventers

When migraine frequency starts to move from episodic to high and then towards chronic, it's time to concentrate even more on prevention.

There are many ways to prevent migraine. Not all involve taking medication. In previous chapters we have considered some self-management strategies you might try. Now we'll focus on some medical treatments, including tablets, neuromodulation devices and injections. We'll also look at the evidence for some alternative therapies, such as acupuncture and biofeedback.

All these options fall under the umbrella 'migraine preventers'. One may work better for you than others. When you speak to your doctor or headache specialist, it will help to know something about the ways in which different preventers work, and why one preventer might be a better fit for you.

When should you use a preventer?

I usually raise the option of adding in a migraine preventer with one of the following scenarios:

- There are more than five attacks per month.
- A series of rescue plans have been tried and aren't working.
- Acute treatments are causing unacceptable side-effects.
- Aura is frequent and troublesome.

Where medication overuse from simple painkillers or triptans could become a problem, I'll often advise trying a preventer in an effort to move the threshold for getting a migraine attack further away. This can help reduce the number of days that a person has to take rescue treatments.

A preventer doesn't prevent migraine attacks from ever happening again. As we saw in Chapter 1, migraine is a lifelong, genetic, neurological disorder. So it's not a realistic goal to expect a 100 per cent reduction in attacks. To be considered effective, a preventer should be reducing the impact of your attacks by about 50 per cent. Your migraine diary will be invaluable for monitoring progress.

People sometimes wrongly assume that, once they have started using a preventer, they must use it for life. This is not the case. If a preventer has succeeded in reducing the irritability of your brain and the impact of your attacks by 50 per cent, it may not be necessary to continue with it.

In my clinic I usually suggest maintaining the effective dose for between six to twelve months. Then, after discussing how quickly to drop the dose and over what period of time, the patient and I may decide to gradually stop it. Most people can do this successfully. If migraine attacks recur later, the preventer can always be prescribed again.

Making the choice

The discussion about which preventer to try is often a long one. This is where having advice from a healthcare professional with specialist training in migraine and headache can be so helpful.

Don't forget to take your migraine diary! You'll need to discuss the details of your symptoms, including the frequency and intensity of your attacks, as well as the treatments you have already tried. Your medical history may also influence the choice. Other factors may include availability and the cost of treatment options where you live.

Together, you and your doctor can begin to consider the effectiveness and side-effects of medications, including rarer things to watch out for. Doctors have to give information about the possible side-effects, but it's not usual to get all of them. So don't let the thought of some side-effects put you off. For many medications, you may not notice any at all.

Currently the best way to find out if a preventer suits you is simply to try it. This trial-and-error method can be frustrating for both patient and doctor, though. In the future we'll hopefully have testing to help us understand a person's genes sufficiently to choose and even tailor a medication to be optimal for them, providing the most effective treatment at the lowest possible dose and with the fewest side-effects. Some pharmacogenetic tests like this are beginning to become available in some places. Until they are more reliable and we build a better understanding of how to interpret their results, trial and error is the best we have.

Medication by mouth

All of the medications that can be taken by mouth to prevent migraine were first developed to treat another condition. Broadly speaking, they fall into four categories:

- **Antidepressants** – to treat mood disorders
- **Anti-epileptics** – to treat seizures
- **Antihypertensives** – to treat high blood pressure
- **Antihistamines** – to treat allergic reactions.

Antidepressants	Anti-epileptics	Antihypertensives	Antihistamines
Amitriptyline Nortriptyline Venlafaxine – a serotonin– norepinephrine reuptake inhibitor (SNRI)	Topiramate Valproic acid (sodium valproate)	Candesartan Propranolol and other beta-blockers	Flunarizine – a calcium channel blocker Pizotifen – a serotonin antagonist

The four classes of common migraine-preventer medications

All of these medications developed for other conditions have some evidence of benefit in migraine prevention. Drugs used for migraine in the past do not appear in the table if, at the time of writing, there is no evidence from studies to prove that they help.

The fact that they are used for these other conditions does not mean a person with migraine must also have one of these conditions to have this medication prescribed. Nor does it mean that you might have one of these conditions because you have migraine. But if you *do* have one of these conditions, that can help you and your doctor or headache specialist decide which one to try first.

The British Association for the Study of Headache (BASH) offers up-to-date, detailed factsheets about preventers on the headache.org.uk website.

You'll need to start with a low dose, increase slowly and stay on the maximum dose you can tolerate for at least three months, before deciding if one of these medications works for you. There is no evidence that taking two different ones at the same time works any better at preventing migraine attacks than trying one at a time.

There is some research into the interesting possibility of using melatonin to prevent migraine attacks, but not enough is yet known about doses, duration, safety or efficacy.[1]

Katerina's story

Katerina had taken her triptan occasionally for years and it worked well. With her busy job and worries about her kids and elderly parents, her migraine attacks had increased recently. She was taking the triptan frequently, often ten days each month. She wasn't sleeping well.

We checked that her lifestyle routine was regular. Magnesium and riboflavin supplements had also helped. We decided to try the antidepressant amitriptyline in a small dose as a preventer. She increased the dose twice before I next saw her. She reported better sleep and her migraine attacks had reduced to one per week. She had a dry mouth and daytime sleepiness in the first two weeks, but these settled. We decided to continue the same dose going forward, with the option to increase the dose in small steps if her migraine attacks weren't controlled well enough after a couple of months.

Medication by injection

There are three types of injections given for migraine today. One delivers antibodies to prevent pain signals; the other two act on key nerves around the face and head.

- **Anti-CGRP monoclonal antibody (mAB) injections**: These are the new kids on the block of migraine prevention. There are currently four in use: fremanezumab, galcanezumab, erenumab and eptinezumab. All target the calcitonin gene-related peptide (CGRP), the key pain-triggering chemical in one of the pathways causing migraine in some people.

  These injections contain antibodies, similar to the ones we naturally produce to fight infection, which are targeted to block the effects of CGRP. They work by attaching either to the surface of the CGRP (ligand) circulating in your body or to the receptors on cells that it fits into. This blocks or dampens the route by which pain signals pass to the brain. It's a bit like trying to stop an electric plug fitting into a socket. You could either put a safety cap into the holes of the socket (the receptor) or a plastic moulded cover on the three prongs of the actual plug (the CGRP ligand). Both approaches would work to stop electricity, or pain signals, from flowing. The pathways in the brain are more complicated than this simple illustration of course. Other pain chemicals may be involved, or may be more significant in generating migraine in certain people.

  The development of these mAB injections has been met with excitement, as they are the first preventive medications designed specifically to work against migraine. They seem to be well tolerated and low in side-effects. If you are prescribed mAB injections, you'll have to inject yourself at home, or get a relative or friend to do it for you, either monthly or every three months, depending on the specific drug chosen. This might sound difficult, but many people – even those who don't like getting jabs – are able to do this quite easily, once taught. Many even enjoy being in control of their treatment in this way. Each dose is quite costly, so there may be restrictions or conditions on their use through your local health service or insurance.

I have prescribed mAB injections for quite a few patients since they became more widely available in the UK in 2018. My patients' feedback has largely been encouraging. Roughly one-third of people describe the treatment as 'life-changing'. Another third get some benefit, with many reporting a 50 per cent reduction in the impact of their migraine attacks.[2] Sadly, there is also a proportion of people in whom mAB injections don't seem to have much effect. Nothing works for everybody.

It is not known how safe these antibodies are to use over the long term, so the current guidance is to use them for a year and then review treatment options with your doctor or headache specialist. By then, we may know more about how effective these are, why they don't work in some people and whether using them long term is safe.

- **Onabotulinum toxin A**: Commonly known as Botox, this neurotoxin created by bacteria was discovered by chance to be helpful for reducing migraine when some people, using it for cosmetic purposes, found that their migraines diminished along with their wrinkles. In the years since, researchers worked out a protocol called PREEMPT for the best doses to use and the best sites to inject.[3] This protocol identifies thirty-one injection sites around the forehead, temples, back of the head, neck and shoulders. Sometimes up to eight additional injections can be given at particularly painful places on the scalp. The injections are repeated regularly, preferably every twelve weeks. The recommendation is to have at least two sets of injections if you are going to try Botox, as some people only see a benefit after the second round. The effectiveness often builds up over time too. Botox is usually well tolerated, although the injections can be quite stinging.

When used for treating migraine, Botox acts on the sensory nerves around the scalp and face, stopping them from sending the signals to the brain that start an attack rolling. When used for treating wrinkles, it acts on the motor nerves that make our facial muscles of expression work. For example, people who have had Botox treatment in the forehead can't raise their eyebrows. The motor and sensory nerves of the face are very close to each other. If Botox injections are not placed accurately, or the person has a slightly different nerve supply to the forehead than the norm, they might experience a drooping or raising in one or both eyebrows. While this may be disconcerting, it wears off after twelve weeks. Botox injections should be done by someone who is properly trained in their use for migraine. Without this training, they could use the wrong dose, or inject too few sites or the wrong sites. Partial treatment can be less effective or can lead to problems.[4]

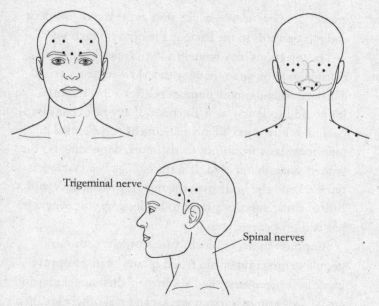

Map of some of the PREEMPT protocol's thirty-one sites for injecting Botox in treating migraine

I have seen some patients in my clinic really benefit from Botox treatment. But, as ever, nothing works for everybody and it is costly. In the UK availability on the NHS is strictly controlled following rules set out by NICE (National Institute for Health and Care Excellence). If you qualify, the clinic that prescribes these injections for you will require you to keep a detailed migraine diary to monitor your response.

- **Nerve blocks**: There are nerves all around the face and head that are implicated in sending pain-triggering messages to the migraine-generating centre in the brain. The most common nerves to be blocked by injection are the two greater occipital nerves, which start at the top of the neck and run upwards to the back of the head on each side.

The injections may contain a local anaesthetic or a combination of anaesthetic with a slow-release steroid. The anaesthetic causes numbness after a few minutes. It's an odd feeling – 'as if the back of my head has disappeared' is how some of my patients have described it. This numbness lasts from four to six hours, depending on the type of anaesthetic used. If a steroid has been added, it is released into the body over the next few weeks. As with Botox, these injections need to be done by someone who has had proper training.

Response to nerve blocks varies widely, with some people getting immediate relief; others having improvement in the frequency and severity of their attacks lasting anywhere from two to ten weeks; and still others seeing no benefit. The injections can be repeated, however, and for some this can improve the response. Your headache specialist will guide you as to how frequently you can have these. Greater occipital nerve blocks can be a good option for women whose migraine attacks have worsened during pregnancy, when it's advised that they avoid treatments that can cross over into the womb through the placenta.

Neuromodulation devices

As we saw in Chapter 7, neuromodulation devices work by generating electrical or magnetic impulses that travel into the brain and disrupt migraine-producing pain pathways.

Two of the devices that have been used to treat acute

migraine attacks, the Cefaly Dual and sTMS mini, have also been helpful in preventing migraine. The Cefaly Dual, which generates electrical impulses to stimulate the supraorbital and supratrochlear nerves, can be used for twenty minutes a day as a preventer. Although it's no longer available at the time of writing, the sTMS mini, which generates magnetic pulses, has also been used as a preventer. Other devices have been trialled but none have so far been useful. Keep an eye out to see if the sTMS mini reappears or if other promising devices using neuromodulation are developed.

Alternative therapies

Now let's look at the alternative therapies that are most often discussed among people with migraine. Some have evidence to suggest they help. Others need more research to prove any benefit.

- **Acupuncture**: A therapy where fine needles are inserted into specific points in the skin, acupuncture has been used as a medical treatment in China for centuries and is now widely used around the world. It is increasingly cited as being helpful in managing pain conditions, including migraine.

  After reviewing many studies, in 2016 Cochrane, a global medical research charity whose mission is providing people with high-quality evidence for making healthcare decisions,[5] concluded that there was moderately good evidence to support the use of acupuncture as a pre-venter for migraine attacks. Their review found that for people who have six days with migraine per month on average, treatment with acupuncture could reduce this to three and a half days. Acupuncture was also more effective than the person's usual care on its own or a placebo of sham acupuncture, where needles are placed at points unrelated to treating pain through acupuncture. However, a similar review of studies by the British Acupuncture Council argued that 'standard' acupuncture is not likely to be helpful for people with migraine because the impact of this condition varies so widely.[6] This echoes my experience in clinic helping patients choose treatments. For any migraine plan to work, it needs to be personalized.

The 'doses' of acupuncture you might receive are not easily standardized. The placing of needles in specific points, the timing of placing and changing the position of needles, the frequency of treatments and your acupuncturist's training and experience can be highly variable.

Although acupuncture seems to be effective in many people and may well be worth trying, the placebo effect must also be considered. In some studies of treatments used for migraine, the placebo effect has been found to be high, with 30–50 per cent of patients reporting an improvement although they were given inert therapies. Sometimes people improve even when they have been *told* that the pills they are taking are dummy pills.

This placebo effect is not necessarily a bad thing, in my opinion. After all, if you feel better for any reason, that's a win. What concerns me is when patients pay money for unproven, untested or potentially unsafe remedies.

These not only give false hope but can also eat into your bank balance, and financial stress worsens mental health. Always bear the placebo effect in mind if you are being asked to pay for a therapy. Ask about the evidence. Find out how many researchers have actually studied the therapy you're considering. Then you can make an informed decision.

- **Daith piercing**: This is a small metal ring placed in the internal cartilage fold of the outer ear, above the ear-canal opening. Anecdotally some people have reported that these piercings helped reduce their migraine attacks, although I have also heard just as many anecdotes from patients in my clinic who have found they had no effect. They were sometimes happy that they had got a cute piercing, though!

The theory is that the piercing hits an acupressure point that is said to be helpful for treating migraine pain. However, there are currently no studies showing this is of benefit,[7] and no evidence to make me suggest you try it. Having any sort of piercing can lead to infection, pain or slow healing of the wound, especially in the ear cartilage. There are some reports of Daith piercings worsening migraine too.

That hasn't stopped a vibrant debate about Daith piercings brewing on social media.[8] This reminds me to acknowledge once again how so many people with migraine are desperate to find something – anything – to help soothe their pain. It's very easy to be persuaded to spend money on an unproven remedy if you've not found anything that works well for you. Remember, migraine is a fluctuating condition. It will naturally ebb and flow in severity.

- **Cannabis therapy:** 'Medical cannabis' is the term used to describe cannabis or its components when prescribed by a doctor for a medical condition. The most common condition for which medical cannabis is used is chronic pain.[9] Cannabis treatment for pain, and in particular headache, has been described from as early as the third and fourth centuries BCE. In her book *Migraine: A History*, Dr Katherine Foxhall described how doctors in the nineteenth century apparently liked to prescribe cannabis, rather than opium, for migraine pain.[10]

  Cannabis was criminalized in the UK in 1928 and in the US in 1937 and remains illegal in many places. Its use has gained a more dubious reputation and stigma. For this reason it's often politically difficult (if not impossible) to research its medical effects. Where studies have been undertaken, the data can be hard to untangle, given the variability inherent in herbal products grown in diverse conditions, as well as a lack of foundational knowledge about dose strengths. Cannabis strains differ in the quantities of cannabinoids, such as CBD (cannabidiol) and THC (Δ^9-tetrahydrocannabinol), and other active chemicals that they contain.[11]

  Medical cannabis can now be prescribed in the UK, some parts of the US and other places for certain conditions, but there is still a lot of work to be done to explore its safe, legal and consistent use as a medication for migraine. At the National Migraine Centre we do not currently recommend it.

- **Biofeedback and relaxation techniques**: These are tools used to train people to exert some control over their autonomic nervous system – the part of the nervous system that controls body functions like the beating of the heart and breathing. Often this involves using an instrument to get a reading of some biological characteristic: for example, skin temperature or muscle tension. You are then taught to observe how these readings change in response to stress-inducing situations and to practise ways to control this. Because the autonomic nervous system is implicated in migraine, biofeedback can be useful in reducing both stress and the impact of attacks.

  Let me give you an illustration. Check your own muscle tension in your neck and shoulders or forehead right now. Are your shoulders creeping up towards your ears? Are your teeth clenched? Do you have a furrowed brow, a constant frown? By becoming aware that these areas of your body are tense, you may be able to slowly breathe out, releasing the tension, imagining it falling down to the floor and away. Just while reading this your facial muscles may have relaxed somewhat.

  With biofeedback, you would connect a device called an electromyogram (EMG) monitor on these muscles. Each time the muscle tension rises, the EMG emits a beep, raising your awareness of what is happening in your body. With practice, many people who use biofeedback devices learn to sense when their muscles are tensing and return them to a relaxed state more of the time, even without wearing the device.

  When we are relaxed, our hands become warmer as

blood vessels dilate and blood flows nearer the skin's surface. If we are frightened or anxious, the reverse happens: our hands may become cold or clammy. Thermal or hand-warming biofeedback uses these changes in temperature to alert people to alterations in their state of tension and to help them relax.

Finally there's progressive muscular relaxation, an exercise where groups of muscles are tightened and then relaxed in turn, as you breathe in and out, moving from the hands up the arms to the shoulders, then the face and then down the torso to the feet. Once the technique becomes familiar, you can relax problem muscle groups individually. Some people find it helpful for sleep problems too.[12]

The American Migraine Foundation suggests that biofeedback and other relaxation techniques can be helpful in reducing migraine frequency and impact, but often work best in conjunction with medications.[13]

• **Osteopathy**: Many of my patients have seen an osteopath along their journey to find help for their migraine. Osteopathic treatment is based on the concept that the smooth functioning of muscles, bones, joints and ligaments is essential for health and well-being. The therapy typically involves massage, pressure and stretching. In the UK osteopaths undergo a long training and are regulated by the General Osteopathic Council.

A review of studies on osteopathic manipulative therapy (OMT) concluded that the evidence was low for using this to treat migraine.[14] However, the researchers could only identify five studies looking at the effectiveness and safety of OMT for migraine. Once again we need more, good-quality research to be able to support people with migraine who are interested in trying a range of alternatives to medication. Lobby for greater investment in migraine research whenever you can and we might learn more.

9. Women and Hormones

Hormones, those biological controllers of our bodies, change throughout our lives, particularly at key times. In women, falling oestrogen levels are the trigger for worse migraine at the end of the monthly menstrual cycle. Why?

At the end of the menstrual cycle, oestrogen levels drop faster in some women with migraine than in those without.[1] This may sensitize the brain to pain-triggering hormones called **prostaglandins**, which are released by the lining of the womb (the endometrium), increasing women's vulnerability to migraine attacks at this time of the month. And women with migraine have a higher incidence of heavy periods, endometriosis and polycystic ovary syndrome (PCOS).[2] Then, during the transition to the menopause (perimenopause), or if removal of the ovaries has been necessary, oestrogen levels also change, which aggravates migraine for some.[3] About 8 per cent of pre-menopausal women and 12 per cent of perimenopausal women report having high-frequency headache. During this time of life 8–13 per cent of women report the new onset of migraine too.[4] Oestrogen levels and the pain-triggering neurochemical calcitonin gene-related peptide (CGRP) are also known to be linked.[5]

In this chapter we'll look at how natural hormonal fluctuations affect people with migraine and at ways to settle oestrogen-triggered brain irritation. Understanding how your hormone cycles affect you may help you work out better migraine-management strategies.

Your menstrual cycle

Many women find their migraine attacks are more intense, more debilitating and last longer around their monthly period. Worsening symptoms may occur before, during or after the bleed. To be classified as **pure menstrual migraine** (PMM), attacks must occur solely around the time of the period.[6] This is quite rare. Instead many women have **menstrually related**

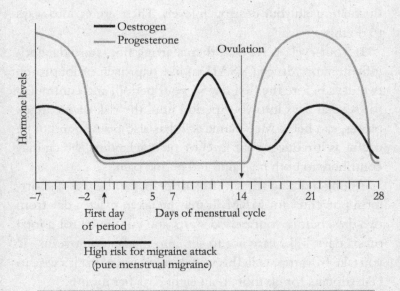

How oestrogen levels fluctuate during the monthly menstrual cycle

migraine (MRM), meaning that attacks are worse around the period but also come at other times in the month.

Oestrogen withdrawal is a trigger for migraine both in the natural menstrual cycle and for some women with migraine without aura who take the combined contraceptive pill. Keeping a migraine diary is invaluable in clearly identifying the patterns in attacks.

Stabilizing oestrogen

If you have MRM attacks that predictably start on or just after your monthly bleed, you may want to try smoothing out fluctuations in your oestrogen levels. There are various ways to do this.

If your cycle is regular, then starting non-steroidal anti-inflammatory drugs (NSAIDs) like naproxen or ibuprofen two days before the first day of your period, and continuing for several days into your period until the risk of an attack passes, can help.[7] Mefenamic acid has also been found to be useful as it reduces your level of prostaglandins, which may contribute to both migraine and period pain.

A longer-acting triptan, frovatriptan, can help as a short-term preventer for MRM. It may be taken twice a day from two days before your period starts and continued for a total of six days. Take care not to slip into medication overuse if you take frovatriptan in this way, remembering that it's wise to take triptans for no more than eight days per month.

Taking a magnesium supplement may also help in MRM (see Chapter 3 for advice about this supplement).

Topical oestrogen gels or patches, previously advised for

use for a few days at the end of the monthly cycle, tend to simply delay the drop in oestrogen and any oestrogen-withdrawal migraine attack.

Contraception

Another way to manipulate your hormone levels is by taking birth-control pills (oral contraceptives). But a word of caution! If you are suffering from migraine with aura, it is not advisable to use a birth-control pill that contains a combination of the hormones oestrogen and progestogen. Migraine with aura seems to bring an added risk of stroke if these 'combined' pills are used.[8] Pills containing just progestogen are safe for people with migraine aura or at risk of stroke, and are very effective as contraceptives. Injected and implanted progestogen contraceptives are safe to use too. Of course other health factors must also be considered when choosing a contraceptive method.

If you have migraine without aura, then you'll have more choices for hormone-based contraception. For MRM without aura, the week with a break from the pill in the 'three weeks on, one week off' pattern advised for years can lead to an oestrogen-withdrawal migraine attack, however. The attacks commonly start in the first four days of the week off the pill and often surge to their highest frequency between days three and six. Taking pill packets consecutively without a break can help control this, and mean you have fewer periods. This is commonly advised in family-planning clinics, although it's not a licensed method. If breakthrough spotting occurs, you simply stop the pill for four days and then restart. Check with your doctor or family-planning adviser before trying this method.

One of the progestogen-only pills, desogestrel, can be used by any woman with migraine who needs contraception. It doesn't increase your risk of cardiovascular side-effects like stroke or heart attacks.[9] This pill seems to be safe and is usually well tolerated, although unpredictable bleeding patterns can be a nuisance. It works for migraine reduction by inhibiting the release of eggs by the ovaries, resulting in a reduction in the hormonal fluctuations that increase the likelihood of a migraine attack.

It's important to know that the preventer topiramate can affect the effectiveness of contraceptive pills, so if you're taking it you could fall pregnant when you had not planned to. Topiramate needs to be used with caution because of this. Another preventer, sodium valproate, can cause birth defects if you become pregnant while taking it. In the UK it's not recommended for use by women and girls with child-bearing potential unless they have followed very strict guidelines set out by the government's valproate pregnancy-prevention programme.[10]

Pregnancy

Pregnancy ushers in big hormonal changes. Some women are so worried about how they will cope with migraine during pregnancy, and then caring for a baby, that they defer getting pregnant and may even decide it's too big a challenge. Yet in 50–75 per cent of women with migraine, pregnancy can be a positive time, with migraine improving and even settling completely. Some women have told me they were even advised by others to get pregnant to help their migraine. This kind of glib remark is not helpful.

Migraine attacks may remain the same in pregnancy as beforehand. However, typically:

- 20 per cent improve in the first three months (trimester).
- 50 per cent improve in the next three months.
- 80 per cent improve in the final three months.[11]

Why exactly migraine improves during pregnancy is not yet fully understood. It may be that because oestrogen levels rise during pregnancy, this reduces the frequency of migraine attacks, in particular in women with migraine without aura or those who had MRM previously. Natural painkillers produced by the body in pregnancy may also help.

Some women – about 8 per cent – find that their migraine symptoms don't improve in pregnancy. Some have aura without headache. About 10–14 per cent of women with migraine with aura report that their attacks started or worsened in pregnancy. One review of studies suggests that 1–10 per cent of women have their first migraine without aura in the first trimester of pregnancy.[12]

It is important to monitor blood pressure closely if your migraine worsens in pregnancy, as there is an increased risk of high blood pressure and pre-eclampsia, a serious condition causing high blood pressure, protein in the urine, leg swelling and sometimes seizures.

After the baby's birth, headache occurs in about 30–40 per cent of all women, and not only in those with migraine. Most of these attacks develop during the first week after delivery, not usually on the day of the baby's birth. Migraine may return quite quickly, when oestrogen levels fall swiftly back to pre-pregnancy levels. Disturbed sleep and the new responsibilities of parenthood don't help, either. About 55 per cent of mothers find their migraines return to the pattern they had before pregnancy about a month after the birth.[13]

If you get a new headache during pregnancy, and have not previously had headaches, it's really important to be sure there are no other reasons for the headache occurring.[14] Headaches can be secondary to more serious conditions in pregnancy, particularly if they start out of the blue. So please see your doctor about any new or unusual headache.

Treating attacks during pregnancy

No researcher will ever get permission to study new treatments in pregnant women and see if the drugs cause harm to the women or babies. So instead the safety of medicines in pregnancy is assessed by collecting data after women who have taken medications during pregnancy, sometimes inadvertently, have given birth. This retrospective data is then collated in a registry.

When treating migraine in pregnancy, the goal is to use the lowest dose of effective medication for the shortest amount of time. All the usual things that help to reduce migraine – regular eating, good sleep quality and relaxation exercises – are a sound, safe start. Keep caffeine intake low, or avoid it completely.

The Best Use of Medicines in Pregnancy (bumps) website[15] gives information about medication use while pregnant.

Always check with your obstetrician and headache specialist if you are uncertain if something is safe to take. Poorly treated attacks can lead to harm through low-quality nutritional intake, interrupted sleep, stress, anxiety and even depression.

Paracetamol (acetaminophen) can be used safely in pregnancy, as it seems to have no effect on the developing foetus. It may not be very effective for migraine pain, however.

Many women ask if they can still use their usual regime of aspirin, NSAIDs, anti-nausea medication or triptans, or some combination of these. Aspirin and NSAIDs such as ibuprofen and naproxen can cause problems in the baby's circulation when it is born. As of 2020, the bumps website states that NSAIDs can be used in the first six months of pregnancy, if needed, but should be avoided in the last three months. There are factsheets about other drugs on their website.

Avoid combination medications that contain more than one active drug ingredient. Many have caffeine, aspirin or codeine in them. Also avoid single-ingredient opioid tablets such as codeine or tramadol. They may affect newborns and can easily lead to medication-overuse headache.

Triptans have been around for years now. Registry data is very reassuring that most of these drugs can safely be used during pregnancy with no evidence of harm to the developing foetus or any increase in birth defects.[16] Shorter-acting triptans, especially sumatriptan, have been looked at in greater detail. There is less information for longer-acting triptans such as frovatriptan and naratriptan.

Nausea and vomiting are often present in pregnancy and, if you are a woman with migraine who also gets nausea or vomiting in your attacks, you may wish to take a safe anti-sickness drug (anti-emetic). Medications that can help migraine-induced nausea and vomiting, such as prochlorperazine, metoclopramide, domperidone and ondansetron, can all be taken in pregnancy, with no concerns currently about their safety.

The supplements magnesium and coenzyme Q10 can usually be taken safely while you're pregnant too, but do check first with your doctor. Riboflavin (vitamin B2) and the herbal products mentioned in Chapter 3 are best avoided during pregnancy.

Preventing migraine in pregnancy

Preventive therapies are sometimes needed in pregnancy. The first choice among the preventer medications discussed in Chapter 8 are the beta-blockers propranolol and metoprolol, which are also used for high blood pressure (antihypertensives) and are safe in pregnancy. These can aggravate asthma, however, so I suggest avoiding them if you have a history of asthma, even just in childhood.

Other antihypertensives, such as candesartan and lisinopril, are not safe in pregnancy. Similarly, the anti-epileptic group of preventers is largely not safe. Sodium valproate, topiramate and gabapentin have been linked with birth defects. Where a beta-blocker can't be used or doesn't work, the antidepressant amitriptyline is recommended.

All preventive medications should be reduced in dose during the final few weeks before delivery, if possible, to minimize the possibility of withdrawal effects on the newborn baby.

Oral steroids like prednisolone have been used for status

migrainosus (prolonged attacks) in pregnancy. However, if these are used, they should be taken in a low dose for a short period.

Greater occipital nerve-block injections seem to be safe too and, if effective, can be particularly useful in the first trimester, when migraine may be more troublesome. The injection may be just a local anaesthetic or the combination of steroid and local anaesthetic. Botox injections may be safe but there is not much data on these, so I currently advise my pregnant patients to avoid them.

The new neuromodulation devices and anti-CGRP drugs have not been studied or used in pregnant women sufficiently for us to know whether they are safe to use. As time goes on, more information about these will become available.

Breastfeeding

Breastfeeding is the best way to nourish your baby, if you're able to do it. It gives a great immunity boost to the baby and reduces the risk of breast cancer in mothers. Breastfeeding also seems to deliver a protective effect in migraine, delaying attacks from returning after giving birth.

Take care with your choice of migraine treatment during breastfeeding, however, because whatever you take may be passed on, to some extent, to your baby in your breast milk. This is especially important in the early months. As your baby gets older, its ability to metabolize drugs will improve, so the risk of transferring medication through the milk is less worrying.[17] In general, if the amount of drug found in breast milk is less than 10 per cent of the dose in the mother, a drug is considered safe.

For acute migraine attacks, paracetamol and ibuprofen are usually the safer, preferred choice among simple painkillers. Avoid aspirin, as there is a small risk that aspirin in breast milk can cause a rare but serious condition called Reye's syndrome in the baby.

The anti-sickness drugs metoclopramide and domperidone can both increase blood levels of prolactin, a hormone needed for breast development and to produce milk. Domperidone is thought to be safe in doses of 30mg per day or less. The European Medicines Agency recommends that domperidone should only be used at the lowest effective dose for the shortest possible duration (less than a week). Prochlorperazine can be used instead, although very young babies may be sedated by it. This creates a risk of their breathing being affected, so caution is called for.

Triptans seem to be safe, with most of the available evidence being about the safe use of sumatriptan.[18] The US Drugs and Lactation Database (LactMed)[19] is very reassuring about using sumatriptan during breastfeeding, with some evidence for eletriptan, rizatriptan and zolmitriptan as well. There is no safety information just yet about almotriptan, frovatriptan or naratriptan, and I'd advise waiting for more data. In the UK the Breastfeeding Network (breastfeedingnetwork. org.uk) is a useful source of information for nursing mothers.[20]

There are many options for migraine preventers for nursing mothers.[21] As in pregnancy, magnesium and coenzyme Q10 can be taken safely. Riboflavin (vitamin B2) can be too. Beta-blockers can also be used, with metoprolol being preferred to propranolol. Amitriptyline and nortriptyline can be used if beta-blockers can't be taken or don't work. Although it should be avoided in pregnancy, candesartan is safe during breast-feeding. One serotonin–norepinephrine reuptake inhibitor (SNRI) antidepressant, venlafaxine, has also been used in nursing mothers with no reported ill effects to the baby.

And both nerve-block and Botox injections appear to be safe when done by an experienced practitioner.

Perimenopause and menopause

The perimenopause – sometimes called the menopausal transition – is the time when ovarian function begins to decline and hormone production gradually stops. Periods often become irregular. This usually starts between the ages of forty and fifty-five and commonly lasts about four years, but can range in duration between several months and ten years. During this time of change, hormone levels become a roller-coaster ride, with dips and surges causing menopausal symptoms to worsen and improve unpredictably. Symptoms may continue for many years after the final menstrual period. A person who has their ovaries surgically removed, or who receives treatments to stop their ovaries from producing oestrogen, will experience a sudden onset of menopause.

Fluctuating hormone levels often coincide with other life changes – for example, children leaving home, responsibility for older relatives and job stresses. Together, these make the perimenopause a high-risk time for worsening migraine. After the menopause, migraine attacks tend to reduce, especially in women with migraine without aura. Women who get migraine with aura may find that their symptoms stay similar or that they get aura without headache as they get older.

Hormone replacement therapy (HRT) can be very helpful for managing migraine. Despite media health scares, menopause experts now report that the benefits of HRT – including improved bone strength, reduced risk of heart disease and reduced risk of some cancers like colon cancer[22] – push the balance of risk/benefit in favour of HRT for many women. Those with a history of oestrogen-receptor breast or ovarian cancer are usually advised to avoid HRT, because of concerns about increasing their risk of recurrence.

If you are perimenopausal you can use the combined birth-control pill (containing both oestrogen and progestogen) as HRT until the age of fifty, as long as you do not have aura or other health issues putting you at greater risk of stroke. Of

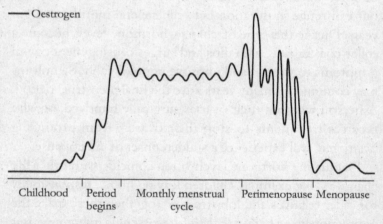

How naturally produced oestrogen levels fluctuate throughout life. Adapted from Lara Briden – The Period Revolutionary, www.larabriden.com.

course this also provides contraceptive protection if you want it. HRT replaces the body's natural oestrogen, so there is no problem with using it after age fifty, even if you have aura.

Topical gels or patches are the preferred delivery method for HRT in migraine because a lower dose can be taken, as it is being directly absorbed through the skin.[23] These also give a more uniform level of hormones, reducing oestrogen swings that trigger migraine. HRT in tablets has to be taken in higher doses as the hormones travel through the gut and to the liver, where they are broken down, leaving less of the dose available.

Gywneth's story

Gwyneth had always had migraine attacks around her period. But she had them at other times too. As she entered her forties her attacks became worse, more frequent and more painful and they lasted longer. She started to get irregular periods, occasional hot flushes and night sweats, which disturbed her sleep. She felt irritable and low. She'd had a Mirena coil fitted for contraception a year before. This contained only progestogen – no oestrogen.

We confirmed that Gwyneth's rescue plan was still helpful, if not as effective as it had once been. To smooth out the fluctuations in her oestrogen levels due to the perimenopause, which I suspected was aggravating her attacks, I suggested some topical oestrogen in the form of a gel to apply to her skin every night. After a few months her migraine attacks had settled down and she was sleeping better and feeling much more positive about life.

Although going through the menopause can be a turbulent time for your brain and body, migraine often gradually improves, with the right advice and treatment.

If you still have your uterus, the lining of the womb can thicken if oestrogen is used on its own. Unchecked, this can lead to a higher risk of endometrial cancer. To avoid this, progestogen must be added to the HRT dose. This can be done in several ways. One option is the levonorgestrel intrauterine system (IUS), or Mirena coil, which has a core containing progestogen that effectively protects the womb lining. Alternatively, some HRT patches and tablets contain progestogen. After hysterectomy, women can use oestrogen-only HRT.

If you are having hot flushes and migraine but don't want to, or can't, take HRT, then the SNRI antidepressant venlafaxine and the selective serotonin reuptake inhibitor (SSRI) antidepressant escitalopram have both been found to help with hot flushes. Improving night sweats may help you sleep better, which can improve migraine too.

All the other preventers can be used with or without HRT during the perimenopause and beyond. An intriguing pilot study found that continuous *testosterone* replacement, by implanting little pellets into fat, seemed to help some women with chronic migraine, but more research is needed to see if this therapy might be helpful.[24]

If you want to learn more about the menopause, Dr Louise Newson's book *Preparing for the Perimenopause and Menopause* (also in the Penguin Life Experts series) is a useful place to start. The British Menopause Society website has information about the perimenopause and the menopause, including a downloadable factsheet to help women and their doctors understand how migraine works during this time.[25] If you are wondering if HRT might improve your migraine, discuss these factors with your doctor or headache specialist, preferably someone with specialist training in HRT and headache.

Transgender individuals and migraine

People transitioning from male to female will use antiandrogens to reduce their male sex characteristics and will take oestrogen to promote female sex characteristics. One study showed that transgender women have a similar occurrence of migraine to cisgender women.[26] Another study found that about one-third of transgender women experienced new headaches or other pain after starting oestrogen therapy, while half of transgender men experienced fewer headaches after starting testosterone therapy.[27]

It is not known why this happens, but it is believed that changing from taking oestrogen orally to a skin patch can help to stabilize hormone levels and reduce attacks in transgender women.

10. Children with Migraine

It still surprises me how often people don't realize that kids get migraine too. Migraine in children and young people is common. It has some similarities to migraine in adults, but also significant differences. Some of the differences in how it manifests can delay diagnosis and cause confusion. Children may get headaches, but these are often shorter and less painful than those in adults. More often kids feel their migraine in their gut, quite literally.[1]

Despite the differences in symptoms, the attacks can be just as debilitating. I have had young migraine patients who have missed a great deal of schooling, been accused of faking their symptoms or been simply ignored. The impact and stigma of migraine can be even worse for kids if their condition goes unrecognized.

A child's experience of migraine

Migraine runs in families. As we saw in Chapter 1, if either parent has migraine, then a child inherits about a 50 per cent risk of experiencing migraine too. If both parents have migraine, this vulnerability is even greater, about 75 per cent.

After I ask patients in my clinic about their family and childhood history, I watch as their eyes light up with recognition. The abdominal pains, vomiting and travel sickness of their childhood now click into place – they are part of their migraine diagnosis. Those who are parents may then see a similar pattern of symptoms in their own children.

About one in ten school-age children has migraine. Though migraine is rare before the age of four, doctors at Great Ormond Street Hospital in London have observed migrainous symptoms such as infantile colic in children as young as eighteen months.[2] Among children with migraine, 50 per cent have their first attack before age twelve. Then, as they enter adolescence, attacks become more frequent. Among those who start having attacks later in childhood, the peak age to first develop migraine is fourteen. These timings are tied to increasing levels of the hormones that trigger growth spurts and sexual maturation.

Before age fourteen, migraine occurs in boys and girls equally. After then, more girls than boys have the condition. Overall, nearly one-third of adolescents with migraine aged fifteen to nineteen get acute attacks. This is a period in life marked by stress – great highs and lows of excitement, arousal, frustration and disappointment.

I find all these figures rather shocking. The debility caused by migraine is bad enough for adults. Imagine the impact on a child or an adolescent trying to deal with these attacks, undiagnosed.

Nearly 50 per cent of children with migraine don't get diagnosed until adulthood. Children with frequent headaches have greater risk of experiencing physical and mental-health problems as well as headache later in life. By age twenty-five, about three-quarters of children with either abdominal or headache-type migraine attacks will have headaches.[3] By age fifty, more than half of them will still have headache attacks.

One study of headache (not specifically migraine) looked at children in secondary school and found that 20 per cent reported having a headache at least once per week.[4] Many of these probably had migraine but it had not been diagnosed. Their headaches negatively affected their lives, both at home and school, on twelve days out of ninety. And children with frequent headaches (two or more per week) scored lower on a quality-of-life scale than children with asthma, diabetes or cancer.

Not making the diagnosis can lead to negative effects for the child, and physical harm too.[5] Roughly 0.8 per cent of children aged twelve to seventeen have chronic migraine, and another 1 per cent have medication-overuse headache. About 5 per cent of children with migraine in one study had unnecessary surgery – removal of a normal appendix – after they described their terrible abdominal pain.[6]

A child or young person whose migraine symptoms are being treated ineffectively or inappropriately, or not at all, will have lower confidence and self-esteem. Anticipatory anxiety, isolation from their peers, loneliness and depression may follow.[7] Stress mounts up as parents are called up by the school about their child's poor attendance. I've even heard of children being punished for complaining about an attack. A child may grow reluctant to go to school, and even refuse to go, as a result. Being labelled as lazy or malingering often causes great distress in a young person who is already struggling with a deeply troublesome physical condition. The impact on their education, social and sporting activities can all damage a young person's well-being.

When should you take your child to the doctor?

If you're now wondering whether your child has migraine, then you've taken the first – and possibly most useful – step towards getting a diagnosis and, from there, finding treatments. You may need to enlist teachers, school nurses, school medical officers, pharmacists, family doctors and specialists such as paediatricians, neurologists and child psychiatrists. Other people may be aware of your child's headache or abdominal pain, especially if they see your child suffering an attack at school. Raising awareness of migraine and how it presents in children is important work.

Take your child to see a doctor if you are in any doubt about the nature or cause of their headaches or abdominal pain, if they are generally unwell or if their symptoms are impacting on their daily activities.

If your child is having any of the following, seek medical advice urgently:

- Fits or blackouts
- Balance or coordination problems
- Onset of headache under age seven
- Unexplained or worsening headaches – more frequent, more severe pain, longer-lasting
- Headache with fever or persistent vomiting
- Personality or behavioural changes
- Poor growth or slow development
- Recent school failure.

What to discuss with your doctor

Kids need to know they are being listened to and properly heard. Personally, I invite children with migraine or suspected migraine to tell me their own story, in their own words and their own way. Their companion, often a parent, only contributes when it feels helpful.

Some kids are initially shy to talk about how they are feeling, but then open up and chat once they gain confidence that their experiences are important in the discussion. Encourage your child not to leave anything out, and let them be the one to lead the conversation. One extremely articulate child who came to my clinic was clearly still aggrieved with a doctor elsewhere who had spoken only to their mother. Your family doctor may already know your child, which may help.

Many of the tools in Chapter 1 for helping you tell the story of your migraine can be adapted for kids. The most useful clues will come from your child's history and pattern of symptoms, just as in the case of adults. Here a simple migraine diary can be very helpful to track symptoms. Some children may prefer to use a 'traffic light' scoring system, rating their bothersome symptoms as green (symptom-free days), amber (problematic, mild symptoms) or red (so bad they had to stop doing things and then took medication or went to bed). This may be much easier to do, particularly for younger children, than rating pain on a ten-point scale. You can also make a simple chart and provide stickers for this. Note down what medications you have given them, along with your sense of whether or not this worked.

Some doctors may ask you and your child to complete the PedMIDAS questionnaire,[8] which helps to assess migraine impact. This simple survey has six main questions; three are about missing or not functioning properly at school, one is about how migraine affects them at home and two are about having to stop activities.

Your doctor will, of course, want to know about the family's history and whether your child has had any of the conditions known to be linked with migraine. These include infantile colic, cyclical vomiting, travel sickness, limb pain, recurrent twisting of the neck muscles causing the head to tilt to one side (benign paroxysmal torticollis) and episodic dizziness (benign paroxysmal positional vertigo, or BPPV).

A main worry may be whether symptoms are secondary to a serious, possibly urgent condition. Blood tests and scans don't help to diagnose migraine, but they can help to exclude certain underlying conditions that cause secondary headaches, if the doctor suspects this. Brain scans are not routinely needed in children with headache, and can unduly raise anxiety levels. The anguish caused by anxiety about a child's health is familiar to most parents and caregivers. This anxiety is very real and needs to be discussed with your doctor.

Symptoms to watch for

Migraine in children and young people causes symptoms both similar to and different from those in adults. Symptoms may also vary by age and by attack. It's believed that in infants head-banging can occur, and that toddlers often become irritable, rocking or crying for no obvious reason.

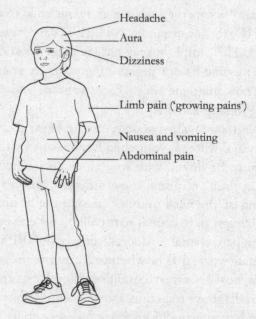

Common migraine symptoms in children and young people.
Adapted from Heather Angus-Leppan, Defne Saatci, Alastair Sutcliffe and Roberto J. Guiloff (2018), 'Abdominal migraine', *BMJ*, 360, art.k179.

- **Lethargy**: In the premonitory phase, before any pain starts, children may feel lethargic, look pale (pallor) or yawn, but they may also have an energy burst.
- **Aura**: Some children describe having visual aura symptoms such as bright spots, blind spots (scotomata), blurred vision or seeing zigzag patterns or coloured, flashing lights. Ask them to draw a picture of what they see, to help them explain. Non-visual aura symptoms may occur too, for example, ringing in the ears (tinnitus),

tingling in the extremities (paraesthesia), light-headedness or, in rare cases, weakness down one side.

If your child is diagnosed with migraine with aura after starting their period (menarche), they should not take oestrogen-containing birth-control pills as there is a small increased risk of stroke with them. Sometimes these pills are offered for controlling troublesome heavy periods that may be associated with migraine.[9]

- **Abdominal pain**: Recurrent abdominal pain is the predominant symptom in some children and adolescents, including those with mild or absent headache. This pain is often central but may move. The child may feel sick or vomit. Some children urinate more frequently or develop diarrhoea during an attack.

- **Headache**: Headaches in children are more commonly on both sides rather than one. They tend to be felt more across the forehead, at the temples, behind the eyes or sometimes over the whole head. Pain is often described as throbbing or pulsating. Attacks can be short, lasting an hour or two, and often resolve completely with simple painkillers and rest in a quiet, dark room.

- **Sensory sensitivities**: Light (photophobia), sound (phonophobia), smell (osmophobia) and touch (allodynia) sensitivities are often present, as they are in adults.

- **Allergy-like symptoms**: Changes to the autonomic nervous system, which controls our automatic body processes such as breathing and heart rate, may cause wateriness of the eyes, a stuffy nose, sweatiness or puffiness in the face.

- **Migraine 'markers'**: A history of 'growing pains' or 'brain freeze' – technically a cold-stimulus headache, where a mouthful of ice cream or another cold food causes pain – may point to a diagnosis of migraine.

In episodic migraine, the child typically recovers completely between attacks. Sadly, in my clinic I have seen some children who have developed high-frequency or chronic migraine. I have also seen children who have been given medications containing codeine, or who have taken painkillers too frequently, and as a result have developed medication-overuse headache.

A treatment plan for their life

Although your child will be dependent on you to help explain their treatment options, it's important to let them guide the choice of treatments and agree to their treatment plan. Start by establishing what their goals and expectations are for treatment. I always aim to fully engage children and young people in the consultation, asking open questions and giving clear explanations. They are the ones struggling with the impact of debilitating attacks. I believe an important factor as to why more than 50 per cent of kids don't stick with their treatments is because they didn't feel involved in the decision-making.[10] If the first treatment they try doesn't work, they feel discouraged. They just want to be like other kids.

Encourage your child to have a regular routine of daily activities. This may feel rather tedious, especially to a teenager who is keen to burn the midnight oil, sleeps in till noon at the weekend and rushes out to school or college with no breakfast. But routine is essential for settling the irritable migraine brain. And with fewer and less severe attacks, they will be able to do more increasingly often.

Triggers for migraine are additive, of course, so reducing anything that is likely to push a child or young person towards an attack at vulnerable times is sensible. I think patients and doctors often underestimate the contribution that some simple changes can make in reducing migraine frequency and severity in kids:

- Never skip meals.
- Eat regular and frequent healthy snacks, including one before bedtime.
- Exercise regularly, and eat and stay hydrated before and afterwards.
- Keep a good, regular sleep routine – that means no long lie-ins.

Stress reduction can help reduce the risk of a migraine attack in kids too. There are lots of ways to approach this. They may enjoy relaxation exercises, such as progressive muscular relaxation or meditations (see Chapter 6). Smartphone apps such as Headspace for Kids, Smiling Mind and Calm may be appealing and useful.

Some may find counselling or psychological support through school, college or local health services to be helpful. Behavioural therapy based on the principles used in **cognitive behavioural therapy** (CBT) has been found to be useful for children.[11] It may be used to give support to the child (and their family) in sticking to their management plan, helping them to remember to take medications in the best way – for example, early in an acute attack as a rescue, and regularly as a preventer. CBT techniques may reduce a child's distress by reframing the way they think about their migraine, allowing them to enjoy life despite migraine and increasing their ability to deal with the pain.

Acute medication

Your child needs a rescue plan for acute attacks that is tailored to their age and size. The timing of this acute treatment, and when to repeat it, should be discussed with your family doctor. Have rescue medication always at the ready, so that your child can take it quickly if they feel an attack starting. This may include the same three key components used in adults: an anti-sickness (anti-emetic) pill such as prochlorperazine; a simple painkiller (NSAID or analgesic) like ibuprofen, naproxen or paracetamol; and a drug specifically designed for migraine (triptan), where needed.

Ibuprofen, at an age-appropriate dose, is recommended as the first-line painkiller in recent guidelines for children and young people. Paracetamol is not very effective for migraine pain in young people, although it can be tried. Adding a triptan can be effective. Triptans are not licensed for children, but headache specialists around the world prescribe them 'off-label' and they are generally considered to be safe. Sumatriptan has been studied the most and has also been found to be effective in adolescents, if used in combination with naproxen. A 2016 Cochrane review of all studies of triptans reported that most of the triptans have been investigated for use in young people.[12] Frovatriptan has been the least studied in kids.

The triptan formulation needs to be chosen carefully. Melt

formulations can be easier to take, and nasal sprays can give rapid relief. But children who are very nauseous or vomit easily may do better with a tablet rather than an unpleasant-tasting melt or nasal spray. Your child's headache specialist should be able to talk through the pros and cons of the options with you and your child.

It's important to know how often the acute treatment can be used per month, as medication-overuse headache does also occur in kids. I normally advise the same rules for children taking triptans as I do for those prescribed to adults: triptans on no more than eight days per month and simple painkillers on no more than fourteen days. Working on a four-week, twenty-eight-day month, these numbers are easy to remember.

I never prescribe opiates or codeine for children with headache, as they can rapidly develop into medication-overuse headache. I would advise avoiding 'combination' painkillers too. Many of those that you can buy at the pharmacy contain caffeine, which is not advisable in children. Caffeine stays in the body for a long time and can impair restorative sleep.

Aspirin should only be used with great caution, particularly in children under sixteen, as it can provoke a rare and very serious condition in children called Reye's syndrome. This can cause brain and liver damage.

Preventers

Your child may benefit from preventive treatment if:

- They have four or more attacks per month.
- They have frequent aura.

- Acute rescue treatments don't work or they are taking them too often.
- Attacks are significantly impairing their day-to-day activities.

As with adults, the realistic goal is to reduce the migraine impact by 50 per cent, not to cure it.[13]

With preventers it pays to 'start low and increase slow', giving time for any side-effects to settle. The maximum dose your child can take without troublesome side-effects should be continued for at least twelve weeks before assessing how well it's working. If the preventer improves things, it can be continued for six to twelve months. After that, the dose should be reduced, or the medication stopped, if possible. Of course if it doesn't help, or side-effects prove problematic, it should be stopped and the plan reviewed.

Preventers for children may include nutraceuticals like magnesium, riboflavin (vitamin B2) and coenzyme Q10. There is sparse evidence and few studies on the use of these in children. Trying one at a time is probably best.

Preventive medications used in adults have also been prescribed for children and young people and can sometimes help. There is a lack of evidence of how well they work in kids, however, and some extra things to consider.

According to one study, propranolol is effective and well tolerated in children. Taking propranolol with cyproheptadine, an anti-allergy (antihistamine) drug, appears to be useful, according to researchers.[14] Propranolol should not be used in children with asthma, however. Cyproheptadine is not licensed for migraine in the UK.

Amitriptyline may also be useful. It is started in small

night-time doses. If side-effects are troublesome, then nortriptyline may be better tolerated.

Topiramate, the only medication currently approved for children by the Food and Drug Administration (FDA) in the US, can improve migraine but unfortunately has some common, unpleasant side-effects, including stomach ache.[15] A 2017 study by the Coalition for Headache and Migraine Patients (CHAMP) reported that both amitriptyline and topiramate were no better in children than taking an inactive placebo.[16] Previous studies had shown a consistent benefit from these, however, and they can be tried.[17]

Cinnarizine is a calcium-channel blocker antihistamine drug that is sometimes used for motion sickness. Like another calcium-channel blocker used in adults, flunarizine, it seems to have benefit in children with migraine. A different type of antihistamine, pizotifen, was widely used in the past to treat migraine in children, but there are no studies proving it works, and it can cause sleepiness and weight gain.[18]

Sodium valproate, an anti-epileptic, might be useful for children, according to recent studies.[19] In the UK it is not given to girls and women of reproductive age.[20]

Melatonin has been used as a preventer and could be useful but more research is needed.[21]

Neuromodulation devices like the Cefaly Dual may be used for children. However, it seems that for these to be effective, they really need a daily commitment of an hour, which may not work for all children. And again there are no studies proving that they work in kids.

Neither nerve-block nor Botox injections are widely used in the UK for children. They have been tried elsewhere, somewhat more commonly in the US. Evidence for their use in children with migraine is lacking, as it has been hard to get approval for studies. Some researchers have looked at using Botox, off-label, in adolescents, and it seems to be safe and well tolerated, but larger studies are needed.[22] Of course these treatments involve having multiple injections, which may make them less viable for children – in my experience, kids aren't keen on getting injections.

When choosing a preventer with your child, take time to talk through the possible benefits and side-effects, keeping in mind their context. Where are they in their schooling? Do they have examinations or other major events coming up? How sporty are they? Are they having anxiety or depression along with migraine? Who will be monitoring their response to the medication, and how? I have sometimes seen teenagers who were about to sit important examinations whose doctor prescribed a preventer that would make them very sleepy or struggle to think straight.

Involving school or college

If your child has migraine attacks on a regular basis, discuss their treatment plan with their school or college. About 10 per cent of twelve- to fifteen-year-olds have headaches bad enough to make them miss seven school days per year.[23] Teachers or lecturers need to understand how migraine is affecting your child, especially if attacks mean they are missing education.

Schools and colleges must identify any particular needs that your child has and work with them, and with you, to make reasonable accommodations to ensure their education proceeds as it would for a child without this disabling condition. Document what has been agreed and ensure that both your child and the relevant teachers and staff are clear about the resulting plan. It should be formally filed and regularly reviewed.

In the UK the Equality Act 2010 protects children with disabling conditions from discrimination, and the Children and Families Act 2014 specifies what schools should do to help. In the US students with disabilities are protected under Section 504 of the Rehabilitation Act 1973. Children with high-frequency or chronic migraine may fall under its remit.

Our children with migraine need better care and understanding of their condition. Much more research is needed too. Educating children and their families about this diagnosis isn't merely about recognizing that a tummy ache might be a migraine attack. It's about tailoring the options for managing attacks to the child's particular needs, explaining what they can expect as they get older and become adults, and telling them about the very real hope for better treatments in the future. The relief on a young person's face when they realize that they are not alone, and that they have power to manage their condition, is one of the greatest rewards for those who treat migraine in kids.

Robert's story

Robert had started getting bad migraine attacks every week, sometimes after football practice, and was missing lots of school. He loved his sports and felt frustrated that he couldn't play. He had seen his family doctor and was taking a migraine preventer, which was really affecting his concentration. He was struggling to study for exams.

When we sat down together, I asked him to walk me through his usual routine. He tended to skip breakfast and was used to lying in bed late on a Saturday to catch up on sleep.

We talked about his sleep routine and trying to keep to a regular schedule of waking, even at weekends. He stopped skipping breakfast and began to pack a protein bar and a drink to have before and after football training. He also added in a bedtime snack of Greek yoghurt with fresh berries. We changed his preventer to find one that didn't affect his ability to study. He was just as pleased as his parents and teachers when he earned a successful set of grades on his exams.

The teen years are an exciting and stressful time of life – but this can also bring on migraine attacks. Creating a routine and finding the right medication can really help young people.

11. Working with Migraine

Under-recognized, underdiagnosed, undertreated, under-resourced and misunderstood – the impact of migraine can affect all aspects of a person's life and ripple out to include family, friends and work. Employment and career pathways can be affected. What are your rights, what help is available and what can you do if you can't work because of migraine?

Should you tell your employer about your migraine?

The decision whether to disclose your migraine is yours. In general, I am in favour of disclosing and discussing migraine with employers as part of a larger effort to improve awareness about the condition. Bear in mind that your employer can't support you through migraine attacks if they don't know your diagnosis. Obviously if you have very occasional attacks, only once or twice a year, you may not feel the need to discuss your condition with them. It's also very unlikely that this level of impairment would fit the criteria for being considered a disability.

Some people are so worried about how their employer will react that they hide that they are a person with migraine. A number of my patients have been reluctant to disclose their migraine diagnosis at work, for fear it will impact negatively on their manager's or employer's opinion of them and possibly damage their career prospects. This can be an issue for actors, dancers and other performers, who may be perceived as unreliable prospects in a fiercely competitive industry. Other professions may restrict treatment options. I have heard, for example, of psychotherapists being told by supervisors that they couldn't try Botox injections, as these could reduce their empathetic facial expressions when seeing clients. I've had patients in the armed forces or security services tell me that they are not allowed to do their job if they take a migraine preventer that is also used to treat depression.

In the UK and some other countries, once you've received a job offer an employer can ask you about your health and sickness records. During this, either you or your employer may ask that you be referred to occupational health services for a report from them. Further review might be needed later to monitor how you are managing. Keep notes of what's discussed or agreed at meetings.

How can your employer support you?

When employers offer a flexible approach and an attitude of trust, people with migraine feel more secure in making better choices to manage their migraine without fear of being penalized. Line managers are crucial here.

Improving the understanding of migraine underpins everything. People with migraine often hear derogatory comments, accusations that they are exaggerating pain and unhelpful suggestions for non-evidence based 'cures'. Respect for migraine as a condition is tarnished by a common attitude that absence from work with migraine means you are probably lazy, malingering or 'pulling a sickie'. We all need to challenge these misconceptions on behalf of everyone with migraine.

We also need to educate our managers and colleagues about the ways in which migraine is a spectrum disease. Understanding that migraine varies widely – not just between individuals, but also within one person over the course of their life – is essential to getting the support you need at work. Many employees have access to occupational health services, but just as many do not and this must be improved.

The Migraine Trust, a UK migraine charity, has developed a downloadable Employment Advocacy Toolkit, to help you discuss migraine and your personal needs with your employer. Similar advice about your rights may be found online from migraine advocacy services worldwide (see Further Reading and Resources on page 211).

Employment, disability and the law

In general, a person is considered disabled by a medical condition if they have an impairment, either physical or mental, that has a 'substantial' and 'long-term' negative impact on their ability to carry out usual activities of daily living (ADL), such as eating, dressing, bathing, toileting, housework and shopping. In any situation where disability is assessed, you may need to provide supporting evidence about your migraine impact, including showing how, without some accommodation, the severity limits your performance in your job.

Disability discrimination is covered by law in many countries. The UN maintains a library of disability laws from around the world.[1] If you have severe attacks or chronic migraine, become familiar with the laws where you live.

In the UK the Health and Safety at Work Act 1974 and the Equality Act 2010 (EQA) outline employers' duties to look after staff and ensure no discrimination occurs in the workplace. The EQA makes the provision that it is the employer's duty to make 'reasonable adjustments' for employees with disabling conditions.

Reasonable adjustments – make a list

The term 'reasonable adjustments' is vague and prone to misinterpretation, often leaving the decision about what is 'reasonable' to the employer's judgement. It is also limited, because sometimes workplaces are impossible to adjust. If you would like your employer to make reasonable adjustments for you, outline the difficulties you encounter. It also behoves you to be reasonable.

Sometimes adjustments can be quite simple. One of my patients had to attend regular briefing sessions, and soon learned these triggered a migraine attack because of habitual glare from the PowerPoint presentation. They raised this with their employer, who arranged printouts of the slides. The result? They got the briefing they needed and happily avoided the trigger.

Common workplace triggers include flickering lighting, poor ventilation, stuffy rooms, colleagues' strong perfume and smells from lunches being prepared in a shared kitchen (fish warmed in microwaves is a trigger, in my experience!). If you're working from home on your own computer, consider if it's suitable for many hours of screen time a day. You can add your personal triggers and sensitivities to this list, then establish what could reasonably be changed to make your work conditions more migraine-friendly. This might include altering shift patterns, if you sometimes work nights.

A list of reasonable adjustments might include:

- Allowing you to go to a quieter, darker private area to rest when an attack starts and you're waiting for your medication to start working.
- Allowing you to work in a less noisy place.
- Flexibility around your working hours, or allowing some home-working, where practical.
- Awareness that flickering fluorescent lights can trigger an attack and may need to be switched off, with alternative lighting arranged.
- Providing anti-glare filters for computer screens.
- Providing blinds or curtains to shield you from sun glare.
- Allowing you to wear protective personal items, such as earplugs or sunglasses, indoors.
- Reducing ambient sounds with noise-cancelling headphones.
- Requesting consideration from other employees about strong fragrances, such as perfumes, or aromatic food in shared lunch facilities.
- Making sure that ventilation and air quality are optimized.

As long as this list is, it's far from exhaustive.

Accommodations may be required for a short period – for example, a month or two – while you're trying, or adjusting, your rescue treatment options. Alternatively you may discover that your overall work patterns aren't functioning well: for example, if night-time shift work, or changing shifts, is unavoidable. In these cases, permanent changes may be called for. Improving work-related stress may be harder to tackle, but may also help.

Employers are not legally obliged to make the suggested changes if they would be detrimental to their business, would disrupt or interfere with usual business operation or cause hardship to the business, or if the change is not possible because of the physical constraints of the work premises. The relative size and financial condition of your employer will also be a factor as to how much they can, or will, adapt your working environment.

A helpful way forward is for you and your employer to discuss together which adjustments you consider to be a priority and how they might be practically implemented. After all, you and your employer are both winners if simple changes result in a happier, healthier, more productive worker! If your employer is not understanding, use the usual route of appeal in the place where you work. If still unsuccessful, you may wish to seek advice from other relevant sources – the human-resources department, senior colleagues, unions, advocacy organizations or perhaps even an employment lawyer, in extreme cases.

Rajesh's story

Rajesh had migraine without aura. He was very sensitive to light glare, air quality, smells and loud noises. His job involved some office work and some site visits. In the office, a colleague loved to douse herself in perfume – a trigger. He also had to hot-desk, often ending up next to a window with the sun shining on his computer screen – another trigger. Onsite, noise could sometimes grow loud and screeching – another trigger. Rushing from place to place, he would snatch a cake bar for lunch, kicking up his glucose (sugar) levels – yet another trigger. When he got an attack, it typically meant leaving work early, and sometimes missing the following day too.

We looked at how his work life was triggering attacks and identified ways to reduce them. Rajesh resolved to take sandwiches with fillings of protein, healthy fats and some vegetables or salad for lunch. He spoke to his boss and negotiated a fixed desk area, away from the window. He approached his colleague about her perfume. She'd not been aware of the problem it was causing him and was mortified, and happy to stop using it on workdays. He was more diligent at wearing the ear defenders provided by his employer onsite.

Modifying your workplace in small but significant ways can be enough to reduce the impact of your migraine. Enlist your employer to help you make the changes you need.

Sickness absence policies

Employment contracts usually contain a section on logging, and dealing with, sickness absence. These may concentrate on processes for monitoring short-term absences. Policies often unduly penalize employees who have a high number of one- or two-day absences to treat migraine attacks. Unfortunately, some of my patients have been called in for disciplinary meetings when their days off sick with migraine started a procedure to investigate their absenteeism. This can be upsetting and feel threatening.

Employers with a good understanding of migraine often adapt this clause to waive counting absence days due to migraine. This enables the person with migraine to relax, removing the pressure to come into work during an attack. Presenteeism (working when not well) can cost employers twice as much as a short absence would. Reducing anxiety about getting an attack can also reduce the likelihood of one occurring – a win/win situation for employee and employer.

If you have had a period of sickness absence due to worsening migraine, a 'return-to-work' planning meeting may help establish whether anything at work was contributing to your attacks and set out a plan to pace your return appropriately.

During discussions like these, your employer will probably want further information or supporting evidence, such as sickness certificates for prolonged absences from your doctor, headache specialist or occupational health department. This can offer a good opportunity to discuss with your clinician the impact your migraine is having on you and ways to optimize your treatment plan. Your health history is confidential, so you must consent to any information about your health being given to your employer by your doctor.

What your employer needs to know about migraine

- It's a genetic, lifelong neurological condition, so it can be managed but not 'cured'.
- People with episodic migraine have fewer than fifteen attacks per month. They are usually well between attacks.
- A person with episodic migraine can develop chronic migraine. People with chronic migraine have more than fifteen attacks per month.
- Attacks and symptoms vary from person to person and throughout life.
- It's not just a headache. Migraine can cause temporary visual changes, dizziness, brain fog, nausea, vomiting, numbness and tingling of the hands and feet, word-finding difficulties and, rarely, temporary paralysis on one side.
- Headache may last anywhere between four hours and three days. You may not be fully back to normal for a couple of days after the headache goes. Awareness of this phase – the postdrome or hangover – is helpful.
- It helps to eat and drink regularly to reduce the risk of starting an attack. Short, frequent breaks support this.

- Attacks can be shortened if you can take medication quickly. Resting for a while in a quiet, darkened place can help too.
- Simple changes in your work environment – for example, to lighting, ventilation or computer screens – can reduce the frequency of your attacks and often aren't expensive.
- Attacks may start quickly, so you may need to be away from work suddenly. Your absence may be short. An employer's sickness absence policy may need to be adaptable to reflect this.
- An employer's support reduces stress, which may reduce the frequency of your attacks and improve your work performance.
- Under the Equality Act 2010 in the UK, and in other countries too, severe migraine can be classed as a disability. Employers are expected to make reasonable adjustments if your migraine reaches this level.

Applying for state benefits

In some cases, work and migraine are incompatible and you may find that you need to apply for state-paid benefits. The state benefits you might be eligible for vary, depending on where you live, your financial status and your tax contribution history. Many countries have strict criteria for proof of disability, and all require supporting evidence. Disability support organizations and advocacy services may be available to explain your entitlements and how to apply. The application forms can sometimes feel overwhelming, so having a family member, friend or other adviser to help you during this form-filling can be a great support. Some people may feel the system is stacked against them, especially if they encounter an assessor who is ill-informed about migraine, seemingly disbelieving or unsympathetic. It's really just bureaucracy at work, so try not to take it personally or become frustrated.

You will need to prove that you are unable to do a full-time job and earn your living because of the impact of migraine. Your migraine diary can be used to confirm the frequency, duration and severity of your attacks. Note down your highest pain score each day, and details about other symptoms and sensitivities that you experience. Charting the impact on daily activities may help your claim too – for example, if you experience debilitating dizziness. Include the type, amount and frequency of medication you use for a rescue plan and for prevention.

You may need a medical report from your doctor or headache specialist listing your medications, past treatments, scans and test results. You may have to describe how well you can manage activities of daily life. Send anything that builds up the full portrait of your migraine attacks. If anyone has seen you during your attacks, a written statement of what they witnessed may be persuasive. The effect of particular work environments, such as the levels of noise or screen glare, should be part of your claim. The assessor may also ask you to consider alternative jobs.

Once all the information for your application is gathered and submitted, there is often a wait while your claim slowly moves forward through the system. You'll probably be asked to attend an interview before the decision is made (in the UK this is called the 'work capability assessment'). If you are turned down, try to find out why. Ask about appeals processes, if you think the decision has been unfair or if you find extra information that might help your claim. It's a long process, but if your claim is finally granted, it will be worth it.

Some organizations that can help you understand your rights and entitlement to benefits are listed in Further Reading and Resources on page 211.

The wider costs

Migraine at work impacts us all as a society. As we saw earlier, the Work Foundation put a price on the huge cost of migraine to the economy: 86 million workdays are lost each year to absenteeism and presenteeism due to migraine in the UK alone, equivalent to £8.8 billion. Adding the direct costs of healthcare brought the total to £9.7 billion each year.[2] If the costs are similar in countries around the world, the global cost of migraine would be in the order of £1 trillion each year. Despite this significant economic impact, migraine is the least publicly funded of all neurological diseases in Europe, and the US National Institutes of Health spent only $28 million on migraine research in 2019 – less than the funding for research on anthrax.[3]

A report published in 2020 by the European Migraine & Headache Alliance looked at the impact of migraine using a questionnaire. The survey found that many employees had no idea of their employer's policy on health and well-being, preventive measures to reduce occupational risks or access to healthcare through their company. About one-third of respondents said that migraine had prevented them taking a job. Sadly, 11.7 per cent reported being fired, and nearly half said they had had job difficulties because of their migraine. The vast majority – 94 per cent – said they felt unable to do their job during a migraine attack. At the same time 60 per cent said they only think of themselves as disabled during attacks, with only 13 per cent saying they feel disabled all the time. My guess is that this last group were people with chronic migraine.[4] These reports confirm what we already know: we need great improvements in how we support people with migraine at work, and we need them urgently.

Thankfully, many employers are now recognizing this and new well-being programmes are being developed by enlightened organizations. The voice of a single person can make a huge difference. After one government employee blogged about her migraine experience at work, the entire UK Civil Service, in partnership with the Migraine Trust, put in place a well-being programme focused specifically on migraine.

It can be well worth approaching your employer to discuss how your workplace can become more migraine-friendly for you and other colleagues with migraine.

12. Migraine Variants

You may have heard different names for different types of migraine. Some of these are distinct subtypes of migraine. Others are old-fashioned terms, no longer used since the updating of the International Classification of Headache Disorders (ICHD-3).[1] Here we'll look at the different subtypes of migraine recognized in the ICHD-3.

Vestibular migraine

Our vestibular system, part of the inner ear, monitors and controls our balance. If it's not functioning properly, vertigo and dizziness result. Vertigo is the sensation that you, or the world around you, is spinning or moving. Dizziness is a looser term often used to describe light-headedness, spinning, faintness or 'wooziness'.

Vestibular migraine (VM) is the most common cause of episodes of vertigo in adults and children. Previously VM was called migraine-associated vertigo or dizziness, migraine-related vestibulopathy or migrainous vertigo.

This vertigo isn't aura. It lasts longer than aura does. About one-third of people with VM have attacks lasting a few minutes. Another third have attacks lasting for hours, and a further third have attacks for days. Some attacks last only a few seconds but occur over and over again, whenever the head is moved or tilted. Visual images may trigger the vertigo – for example, watching a fast-moving train go past or looking at strongly contrasting patterns like stripes, especially if they are distorted.

Despite vertigo being a common symptom in migraine attacks, VM is still underdiagnosed. Dizzy people may be referred to an ear, nose and throat (ENT) specialist or a neurologist, accounting for about 7 per cent of patients in ENT clinics and about 9 per cent of people in headache clinics.[2] Many people with this type of migraine may have hearing and balance tests or scans before a diagnosis of VM is made.

You may have VM if you've had at least five episodes of moderate to severe vertigo lasting between five minutes and seventy-two hours and you have a current or past diagnosis of migraine (with or without aura).[3] At least half your episodes must also have either headache, visual aura or sensitivity to light (photophobia) or sound (phonophobia).[4] Not everyone with VM gets a headache, and this is often the cause for confusion and delay around the diagnosis.

VM can occur at any age but often starts after a long history of other types of migraine attacks. It's more common in women, and attacks that typically include headache may change to isolated vertigo attacks after the menopause. As with all migraine, symptoms may alter from attack to attack and throughout life.

The vertigo can be intense and recurring. Patients in my clinic have described the sensation as being on board ship in a choppy sea, with the deck lurching and falling beneath them. Others tell me they need to grab furniture to stop themselves falling. One young patient had extreme anxiety about getting an attack in the night because they had such difficulty getting out of their bedroom for help. It can have a huge impact on life. Some symptoms occur that are also seen in other vestibular conditions: a feeling of pressure in the ear, nausea, vomiting, temporary hearing loss, temporary hearing changes, travel sickness and, sometimes, sudden collapse.

Another cause of dizziness, Ménière's disease, can lead to progressive hearing loss, however. Ménière's disease seems to be linked to VM and the two conditions show some overlap. It may be hard to distinguish between them in the early stages. Some people with a Ménière's diagnosis actually have VM.

Treatment of VM follows the same principles as treatment for migraine with or without aura, but there are a couple of things to note. Stopping caffeine completely seems to be helpful in VM. In one study, 14 per cent of VM patients found it helped their attacks.[5] Not many studies have been done looking at medication specifically for VM. Triptans, often so useful in reducing headache, don't help much with vertigo, unfortunately. It is fine to try them, though, if you have VM with troublesome headache.

One therapy to consider is **vestibular rehabilitation**, sometimes called 'balance retraining'. If you are referred for balance retraining, you'll need to attend a specialist physiotherapy clinic, sometimes for a few weeks, to learn exercises, including ones for eye movement and posture. You'll need to practise these daily at home. One study found that these programmes could reduce headache as well as anxiety and depression related to VM.[6] If you're diagnosed with VM, ask about being referred to a specialist vestibular physiotherapist.

Hemiplegic migraine

Hemiplegic migraine (HM) is a rare variant of migraine with aura. Two types have been described: familial (FHM), with a clear family history, and sporadic (SHM), where no first- or second-degree relatives are known to have the condition.[7]

'Hemiplegia' is total or partial paralysis of one side of the body. A person with hemiplegia cannot move the affected part. You may have HM if you've had at least two attacks of hemiplegia with fully reversible muscle weakness of the face, arm, hand, leg or foot, or a combination of these areas, along with fully reversible sensory disturbances, such as problems with vision or language.[8]

Weakness tends to progress over the course of twenty to thirty minutes from one part of the body, usually starting in the hand and gradually spreading up towards the face on the same side. During attacks the weakness can switch sides and, rarely, both sides can be affected simultaneously. The affected side may change from attack to attack. Muscle weakness doesn't necessarily happen in every attack but, when it does, it's fully reversible and usually lasts under seventy-two hours. In rare cases it can continue for weeks. Visual disturbances and other types of aura symptoms, numbness, tingling, staggering gait (ataxia), lethargy and fever can all occur too.

If you're wondering if your attacks are HM, pay attention to whether you're truly unable to move your muscles, or your limb feels very heavy but *can* move. It's important to distinguish between actual muscle weakness (motor paralysis) and the sensation of heaviness (sensory loss), which often occurs with aura. This distinction, when not clarified, has led to some people mistakenly being told they have HM when they don't.

Many of my patients with HM have told me that in their first attack, or where aura symptoms came on very rapidly, they worried they were having a stroke or transient ischaemic attack (TIA or 'mini-stroke'). Quite a few had been admitted urgently to a hospital stroke unit for specialist tests. Being rushed into a stroke unit can be distressing, but these conditions need to be excluded.

Four specific genetic subtypes have been identified in FHM. These attacks almost always lead to headache, which can start during the aura or afterwards. Sometimes altered consciousness (even coma), confusion and fever occur too. An attack may be triggered by a quite minor head trauma. I saw a young patient where a small bump on their head was enough to trigger debilitating symptoms of hemiplegia and confusion lasting several weeks. FHM attacks often start in youth, with the average age of onset being between twelve and seventeen years of age. Women are three times more likely to have FHM than men.

Treatment of HM is similar to that for other migraine attacks with aura, but using triptans for them has been controversial. Previously doctors thought triptans might aggravate HM symptoms because they constrict the blood vessels, including those in the brain, but I know many headache specialists who are reassuring about their safety. It is best to check with your own headache specialist about this, particularly if you have any other risk factors. You'll also want to explore preventive treatment options to reduce the impact of these alarming attacks. One patient told me that having acupuncture as soon as motor weakness started helped to shorten their attacks. They were lucky to have a work colleague who practised acupuncture who was often around when attacks came, but getting needling at short notice isn't practical for many.

Retinal migraine

If you have visual aura only in one eye, you have retinal migraine (RM), previously known as ocular migraine. In RM you may have flashes or sparkling lights, blind spots (scotomata) or even blindness in the affected eye, but vision in your other eye remains normal. The loss or change of vision is fully reversible. Changes may spread gradually and can last from five to sixty minutes. They are then followed by headache.[9]

The monocular nature of RM makes this type different from typical visual aura symptoms, which occur in both eyes (see Chapter 2 for a fuller description of aura). You can test this yourself, by closing one eye at a time and seeing if your visual symptoms only affect one side. A specialist can plot changes in your field of vision during an attack.

Treatment for RM is largely the same as for migraine with aura.

Typical aura without headache

With the ICHD-3, the terms 'silent migraine' or 'acephalgic migraine' have been changed to 'typical aura without headache'.[10] This name gives a much clearer description of this type of attack, although isn't so catchy. Basically, if you experience a typical aura but do not then develop headache, you have this. You may have this type in some or all of your attacks.

However, when a person's vision changes and they don't have obvious clues to the diagnosis of migraine, this needs to be investigated to exclude other conditions with similar symptoms. TIAs, or 'mini-strokes', can cause a short disturbance of vision similar to this. If visual symptoms that seem like aura continue for more than an hour, or you have vision loss without aura features or you start having these symptoms for the first time after age forty, consult a doctor or headache specialist to investigate what's happening.

Migraine with brainstem aura

This type of migraine, previously called basilar or basilar-type migraine, is quite rare. There has been some debate about whether it's a separate subtype, but the ICHD-3 classification has it as one for now.[11] Symptoms arise in the brainstem and affect both sides of the body at the same time. To be diagnosed with this subtype[12] you must have at least two of the following:

- Double vision or visual changes in both eyes
- Difficulty in speaking by slurring words (dysarthria)
- Problems with hearing
- Tingling in the hands and feet (paraesthesia) on both sides
- Dizziness
- An illusion of moving (vertigo)
- Ringing in the ears (tinnitus)
- Fainting (syncope)
- Altered consciousness
- A staggering walk (ataxia)

The symptoms should not include weakness of the muscles (motor weakness). Often people who get these brainstem-aura symptoms also get migraine with a more typical visual aura.

If the first attack starts after age fifty, then a full medical assessment, including an MRI scan, is called for to rule out other conditions. There are currently no treatments specifically targeted at this migraine type. For treatment purposes, it can be approached in the same way as migraine with typical aura.[13]

13. Cluster and Other Headaches

Some headache conditions may be misdiagnosed as migraine. However, treatments for these are very different, so it's important to be aware of them – especially those that require urgent or emergency medical attention, such as giant cell arteritis and thunderclap headache.

Primary headaches

These conditions, where headache has not been caused by an underlying condition, include a number of rarer headache types.[1] Among them, cluster headache is a crucial diagnosis to get right. Other primary headache types include hypnic headache, primary stabbing headache and headaches associated with cough, exercise, sexual activity or cold stimulus.

- **Cluster headache (CH)**: One of the most painful headache conditions known, CH is the most common of the so-called trigeminal autonomic cephalalgias (TACs), a group of rarer headache conditions characterized by severe pain and symptoms affecting the autonomic nervous system, which controls automatic functions like breathing and heart rate. People with CH have attacks of intense, excruciating pain, often at regular, predictable times – that why it's sometimes called the 'alarm-clock headache'. More ominously, it's also called the 'suicide headache' because the pain intensity and recurrent attacks lead some people to despair.[2]

I hear distressing stories from CH patients who have struggled to get a diagnosis and then effective treatment. A review of studies found that it takes from one to nine years after a person's first attack for this condition to be diagnosed.[3] With or without a diagnosis, some people have been given medications for migraine by doctors who incorrectly assumed their excruciating headaches would be relieved by standard migraine treatments.

Pain is exclusively one-sided or side-locked. It is often felt in, above or behind the eye or at the temple. Autonomic symptoms accompanying these attacks may include watering and redness of the eye, drooping or puffiness of the eyelid, runny or stuffy nose, redness of the cheek, facial flushing or increased sweating on the affected side. People with CH typically become agitated during attacks and pace up and down, or rock backwards and forwards to try to escape the pain. I've heard of CH patients who have hurt themselves – for example, by punching their head or even pulling out their own teeth to try to distract themselves from the pain.[4]

A history of extreme restlessness can aid diagnosis; during migraine attacks, most people want to stay very still.

Bouts of episodic cluster headache (ECH) may last from weeks to several months. Once the bout settles, there may be a period of time lasting a few months to several years when the person is completely free of attacks. A quarter of patients only ever have one bout. Often bouts are seasonal, being triggered more near the spring and

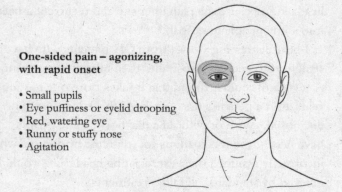

One-sided pain – agonizing, with rapid onset

- Small pupils
- Eye puffiness or eyelid drooping
- Red, watering eye
- Runny or stuffy nose
- Agitation

Some key features of cluster headache

autumn equinoxes. Each single attack lasts between fifteen minutes and three hours, but there can be many attacks over twenty-four hours.

Chronic cluster headache (CCH) is a condition where periods of remission between bouts shorten, so there is no break.

People usually start getting CH between the ages of twenty and forty, but it can occur in children too. More men are affected than women – three to one – another difference from migraine. Sadly, I have also heard that women with CH are sometimes dismissed with 'Women don't get cluster headache.' This is so wrong. They do. My female cluster patients can confirm it! Unfortunately the two diagnoses can also coexist. I have some patients with migraine who later developed CH symptoms.

If you think you have CH or have been diagnosed with it, I recommend OUCH (UK), the Organisation for the Understanding of Cluster Headache (ouchuk.org), which can help you understand this condition and get appropriate support. Gold-standard treatments for acute attacks are high-flow oxygen, which can relieve CH pain in less than fifteen minutes, and sumatriptan injections. Both are expensive. In the UK many people struggle to get these prescribed on the NHS, despite clear guidelines by NICE to provide them.[5] Elsewhere, insurance companies are not always prepared to cover the costs. Battling against these obstacles leads to continued attacks of excruciating pain, unnecessary anxiety and sometimes depression.

- **Tension-type headache (TTH)**: Many people with migraine are told they have tension-type headache. The two conditions can be distinguished, however. TTH is largely featureless. The pain has a pressing or tightening quality and, unlike migraine, is not aggravated by normal movement like walking or going upstairs. Sensitivities to light (photophobia) and sound (phonophobia) are not usually present, and vomiting is unusual. TTH is usually painful on both sides of the head, or feels like a band around the head. Some people with TTH report tenderness around the scalp, but this can also be felt in other headache types. Although it's widely thought to be a common type of headache, TTH is greatly overdiagnosed. Many people who actually have migraine are misdiagnosed with TTH. If you're diagnosed with TTH and experience symptoms of migraine, ask questions.

Secondary headaches

These are headaches attributed to an underlying disease process or medical condition, such as headache caused by infection, tumours, trauma or use or withdrawal from some substances, for example, alcohol, nitric oxide, caffeine and opioids. Below I highlight some of the more important ones to know about. Some are medical emergencies. Others are commonly confused with migraine.

- **Cervicogenic headache**: This is a headache caused by neck (cervical spine) problems, although there may not be neck pain.[6] Trouble with the bones, joints or soft tissues of the neck can cause it. Confusion with migraine occurs because pain messages from the neck and shoulders can trigger migraine attacks, and pain from a migraine attack may also travel downwards from the head to the neck and shoulders. Good attention to posture and a referral to a rheumatologist or physiotherapist may help if this headache is suspected.

- **CSF leak**: Cerebrospinal fluid (CSF) is the cushioning fluid surrounding the brain and spinal cord. Anything that causes a leak and loss of CSF[7] – for example, following a lumbar puncture or epidural – can lead to a headache. A leak can also happen spontaneously. It's a sudden headache, often initially relieved by lying down. It worsens any time the person stands up for a while. Scans to look for the leak may be done, but it's often difficult to pinpoint the leak site as the body may already have repaired the hole. Postural symptoms can change over time, adding to the confusion. Take note of any postural differences in your headache symptoms.

Some people with headaches caused by spontaneous CSF leaks may have an inherited genetic condition called Ehlers–Danlos syndrome, which causes their connective tissues (collagen) to be weaker than normal.[8] This can easily be missed or misdiagnosed.

- **Giant cell arteritis (GCA)**: If untreated, GCA can lead to loss of vision that may be permanent. It must be treated quickly. A simple blood test to check for inflammation should be done urgently, and steroid medication started to protect the eyesight while waiting for a more definitive diagnosis by temporal artery biopsy.

  GCA is an inflammation of blood vessels (vasculitis) that causes a headache with tenderness over the arteries at the temples (temporal arteries). It's more common in people over the age of fifty. It's rare, with only about 1 in 10,000 people in the UK diagnosed with it. It can also bring fatigue, weight loss, fever and loss of appetite. It's linked with polymyalgia rheumatica, which can cause pain and stiffness in the shoulders and legs.

- **Idiopathic intracranial hypertension (IIH)**: 'Idiopathic' means the cause is unknown. 'Intracranial hypertension' means that pressure is raised inside the skull. Diagnosis of this headache is becoming more prevalent, although it's still rare.[9] It's troublesome to treat, but many of its symptoms overlap with other headache conditions, including migraine.

  IIH gives a variable headache, often severe and debilitating, and is sometimes associated with sight-threatening changes in the brain. The headache may worsen if pressure inside the skull increases temporarily, for example, with coughing, straining or lying down. Pounding noises in the ears may be heard (pulsatile tinnitus). It can mimic brain-tumour symptoms and for that reason is sometimes called pseudotumor cerebri (false tumour of the brain).

The raised pressure in the brain is due to too much CSF building up. The pressure on the brain and the nerves from the eyes to the brain (optic nerves) can lead to temporary or even permanent blindness, if not corrected. When a doctor or optician examines the back of the eyes of a person with IIH, swelling of these optic nerves may be seen (papilloedema).

Risk of IIH is higher in girls and women and in people who are overweight or obese. It's mostly seen in women aged twenty to fifty years. Weight loss, medications and sometimes surgery to reduce the pressure have been tried, to manage this condition. Regular eye checks are important, so patients are often seen by both a neurologist and an ophthalmologist (specialist eye doctor).

- **Thunderclap headache**: This is any very sudden-onset headache – a dramatic, instantaneous onset of severe pain, peaking within about sixty seconds.[10] People liken it to being 'hit on the head with a baseball bat' and describe it as 'the worst headache I've ever had in my life'. Urgent assessment in the emergency department is vital.

It is associated with swelling and rupture of blood vessels within the brain (aneurysm), a bleed from which may be life-threatening (subarachnoid haemorrhage).

Scans and lumbar puncture help doctors look for a bleed in the brain. If a bleed is the cause, surgery may be needed to prevent further bleeding.

Clots (thrombosis) in brain blood vessels, temporary spasm of blood vessels (reversible cerebral vasoconstriction syndrome, or RCVS) and other conditions may also result in this type of headache. Sexual-activity headaches can mimic thunderclaps but are not usually dangerous. Embarrassment may make people delay seeking help if they experience headaches during sex. They still need to be checked out, though.

It is very important not to ignore a thunderclap headache. Seek help as a medical emergency, even if you have a history of migraine.

- **Tumours**: People with bad headaches are often very concerned about brain tumours and ask me if they need scans or further tests to exclude these. Migraine is much more common than brain tumours, however.[11]

The headaches from brain tumours tend to worsen gradually over time. They are often worse in the morning and on coughing or straining, and painkillers often don't help much. Pressure in the head from the tumour growing and squeezing the brain can cause headaches, but most people with brain tumours also have other noticeable symptoms, including fits, nausea, vomiting, persistent drowsiness, memory or personality changes, progressive weakness on one side of the body and vision or speech problems. These tend to worsen gradually. It's really important to see your doctor if you are experiencing any of these symptoms occurring with your headaches.

- **Visual snow**: This condition is not a headache, although it's mentioned in the ICHD-3 classification[12] and is commonly mistaken for migraine aura. Sufferers often have migraine too. The main symptom is a continuous visual disturbance over the whole field of vision. Patients sometimes describe it as looking like 'interference or static on a television screen'. Tiny dots flicker in front of the person's vision and overlie the background. Usually these dots are black and white, but they may be coloured or even transparent.

  Up to 75 per cent of people with this also have other visual disturbances:

  - Perceptions of trailing images across the vision as the eyes move, or stationary images remaining (palinopsia).
  - Difficulty in seeing in dim light (nyctalopia).
  - Seeing floaters, flashes of light or coloured clouds or waves when the eyes are closed in the dark (self-lighting of the eye).[13]
  - Many people with visual snow also have ringing in the ears (tinnitus).

    It is the recurring, pervasive and debilitating aspect of the symptoms, despite completely normal eyes and optic nerves, that make visual snow so troublesome. Unfortunately, no good treatments are yet known to help, and further research is needed.

14. Managing Your Migraine

The best way to manage your migraine is to develop a good working relationship with a group of people whom you might think of as your 'migraine advisory team'. So who do you want on your team and how can you help them to help you?

In my clinic, and from my own personal experience as a person with migraine, it seems the first line of support comprises family members and friends, especially if these individuals have migraine themselves and some personal experience of coping with it. When simple measures fail, pharmacists are frequently the next advisers. Many pharmacists have a wealth of knowledge of health conditions and the optimal use of medications to treat them. They know remedies that can be easily obtained without needing a doctor to prescribe them, and can advise on interactions with other medicines you are taking. They can also signpost you to support organizations. These are all very helpful. In my opinion, however, there are rather too many opioid- and codeine-based medications available without a prescription, and I would like to see more cautions around their use in people with migraine.

When migraine symptoms become troublesome, your search for support may widen. Many of the patients who see me at the National Migraine Centre have previously attended appointments with their GP, with doctors who specialize in ear, nose and throat (ENT) conditions, with eye specialists (ophthalmologists), opticians, physiotherapists, osteopaths, acupuncturists and massage therapists.

A surprising number of people with migraine[1] – in some studies nearly 60 per cent – do not seek medical help. Not asking for help is one of the biggest barriers to good care for migraine.[2] Better education about migraine would help reduce the number of people who struggle on, putting up with migraine attacks unnecessarily.

If you seek help from your family doctor, they will need to confirm your diagnosis and then start to develop a personalized treatment plan with you. This can always be adapted along the way, with referrals for more specialist advice being done if necessary. If plan A doesn't work, there is usually a plan B, and a plan C and D.

What are you hoping for?

It's important to prepare for your consultation by thinking about what you hope to get out of it. What patients want does not always match up with what their doctors think they want, according to studies on patient expectations going into migraine consultations. On a basic level, most people want their symptoms reduced as soon as possible, but which symptoms they want controlled may not be so obvious. And about 25 per cent of patients go to their doctor hoping for a cure.[3] This is an impossible goal at the moment, but who knows what research will achieve in the future?

In one study, people with migraine were asked, 'What is the most bothersome symptom of your migraine attack?'[4] It's a great question, because it quickly establishes whether headache, dizziness, brain fog or something else is the most pressing symptom – the one you want and need to minimize as the first priority. Studies often consider a drug to be effective if it provides a 'reduction of headache at two hours'. This may not be what you, as a patient, are most interested in achieving. Patients sometimes tell me, for example, 'I can deal with the headache, but it's the aura [or the dizziness, or the brain fog] that is more of a nuisance.' Knowing your answer to the question 'What is the most bothersome symptom of your migraine attack?' will help to focus the conversation you have with your doctor.

Researchers also asked about patients' expectations for the effectiveness of medications. People said they wanted medications to: 1) take their headache away quickly; 2) stop the attack; 3) prevent a relapse from happening; and 4) let them function normally once more. Those all seem very reasonable expectations to me.

Your doctor has limited time with you, so being organized and prepared with relevant information can be a huge help. I find it useful to hear a patient's recent history first and then go back over their past history, to fill in the background details that I need to make an assessment. If you can, take details with you of any previous medications you have tried, including the doses you took and the duration of the course. Blood-test results and scans that you have already had, plus copies of any previous reports from other doctors, can be very useful too.

Arming yourself with information

When you see your doctor or headache specialist, be sure to bring your migraine diary. You'll also need to be prepared to discuss the following:

- The story of your migraine so far: symptoms, frequency of attacks, severity of attacks and impact of attacks; any observations of triggers you've noticed.
- Your medication history: current and past medications for migraine; current medications for other conditions and drug allergies.
- Your medical history: current and past medical conditions, both physical and mental, and any family history.
- Your personal situation: whatever is relevant – sources of stress, sleep cycles, your occupation, your dependants, the impact of your attacks on your family and job.

Setting your goals
Think about your answers to these questions before seeing your doctor:

- What are you hoping for from the consultation?
- What is the most bothersome symptom of your migraine?
- What action do you want the doctor to take – diagnose, explain, reassure, treat, refer or something else?
- If acute medication is suggested, what are your priorities and goals for a rescue plan? Consider things like the speed of controlling symptoms, helping specific problems such as nausea or dizziness or keeping pain from rebounding.

- **If preventive treatment is suggested, what are your priorities and goals? Consider things like reducing the frequency of attacks, avoiding side-effects or safety with other medications that you take.**

Some doctors may wish to concentrate on talking about medication options with you, but these may not be your priority. In one study, people with migraine were surveyed about their satisfaction with their care. Doctors attending a specialist meeting about headache were asked to predict what the patients valued highly. Some doctors were surprised to learn that what patients valued most in their doctor was a willingness to answer their questions.[5] Next on the list, they wanted doctors to teach them about the cause and treatment of migraine, and how to avoid their attacks.

Make a list of your questions before your consultation and bring them with you. It's easy to forget something and it may be some time before your next appointment. Help your doctor to help you find answers together.

Why now?

It may be helpful to tell your doctor why you are seeking help now. What has made you feel you need more advice at this stage? You might be planning a pregnancy, starting a new job or have a period of exams coming up. Or you may have heard of new advances in treatment, want a second opinion or wish to learn more about a therapy you might like to try. You might even have been nudged, persuaded or cajoled by concerned family members, friends or colleagues because your attacks are getting worse. I've heard this over and over again in my clinic: 'My wife made me come', 'It's affecting my work', 'I might lose my job', 'I can't do my sport at the weekends', 'I keep missing out on things.'

Whatever your reason for seeking help now, to make the most of your partnership with your migraine adviser, the relationship needs to be one of listening, shared discussion and planning.

Managing your migraine

1. **You are not to blame.** Migraine is a genetic, neurological brain disorder. It's not your fault.

2. **You are not alone.** Migraine is very, very common. One in seven people gets it.

3. **You can take control.** Eat regularly. Don't skip meals. Have good sleep routines. Try to exercise regularly. Manage your stress.

4. **You have tools.** Take rescue medication early to improve your chances of stopping an acute attack.

5. **You are a migraine detective.** Track your attacks with a migraine diary to help understand your triggers.

6. **You can take care.** Count the days you take your rescue treatments. Don't overuse them.

7. **You can ask for help.** Preventing migraine attacks helps reduce them in the future. Ask about prevention.

8. **You can be the expert.** Migraine preventers come in many forms – lifestyle, medications, injections, neuromodulation devices. Learn about them.

9. **You can keep trying.** You probably haven't tried everything, even if it feels as if you have.

10. **You can be hopeful.** New treatments are being developed.

Notes

Introduction

1　GBD 2016 Headache Collaborators (2018), 'Global, regional, and national burden of migraine and tension-type headache, 1990–2016: A systematic analysis for the Global Burden of Disease Study 2016', *The Lancet*, doi.org/10.1016/S1474-4422(18)30322-3

2　Ibid.

3　Work Foundation (2018), 'Society's headache: The socioeconomic impact of migraine', www.lancaster.ac.uk/media/lancaster-university/content-assets/documents/lums/work-foundation/SocietysHeadacheTheSocioeconomic impactofmigraine.pdf

4　Rebecca Burch, Paul Rizzoli and Elizabeth Loder (2018), 'The prevalence and impact of migraine and severe headache in the United States: Figures and trends from government health studies', *Headache*, 58 (4), pp.496–505

5　L. M. Bloudek, M. Stokes, D. C. Buse et al. (2012), 'Cost of healthcare for patients with migraine in five European countries: Results from the International Burden of Migraine Study (IBMS)', *Journal of Headache and Pain*, 13 (5), pp.361–78, www.ncbi.nlm.nih.gov/pmc/articles/PMC3381065

6　GBD 2016 Headache Collaborators (2018), 'Global, regional, and national burden of migraine and tension-type headache'

7　Michael Bjørn Russell, Vibeke Ulrich, Morten Gervil and Jes Olesen (2002), 'Migraine without aura and migraine with aura are distinct disorders: A population-based twin survey', *Headache*, 42 (5), pp.332–6, pubmed.ncbi.nlm.nih.gov/12047331

8　Katherine Foxhall (2019), *Migraine: A History* (Baltimore: Johns Hopkins University Press)

1. Are You a Person with Migraine?

1　Stewart J. Tepper, Carl G. H. Dahlöf, Andrew Dowson et al. (2004), 'Prevalence and diagnosis of migraine in patients consulting their physician with a complaint of headache: Data from the Landmark Study', *Headache*, 44 (9), pp.856–64, pubmed.ncbi.nlm.nih.gov/15447694

2　Jyoti Mani and Shailender Madani (2018), 'Pediatric abdominal migraine: Current perspectives on a lesser known entity', *Pediatric Health, Medicine and Therapeutics*, 8, pp.47–58, www.ncbi.nlm.nih.gov/pmc/articles/PMC5923275

3 Stephanie S. Faubion, Pelin Batur and Anne H. Calhoun (2018), 'Migraine throughout the female reproductive life cycle', *Mayo Clinic Proceedings*, 93 (5), pp.639–45, doi.org/10.1016/j.mayocp.2017.11.027

4 GBD 2016 Headache Collaborators (2018), 'Global, regional, and national burden of migraine and tension-type headache'

5 Padhraig Gormley, Verneri Anttila, Bendik S. Winsvold et al. (2016), 'Meta-analysis of 375,000 individuals identifies 38 susceptibility loci for migraine', *Nature Genetics*, 48 (8), pp.856–66, pubmed.ncbi.nlm.nih.gov/27322543

2. Understanding Phases and Triggers

1 Todd J. Schwedt and Catherine D. Chong (2015), 'Functional imaging and migraine: New connections?', *Current Opinion in Neurology*, 28 (3), pp.265–70, www.ncbi.nlm.nih.gov/pmc/articles/PMC4414904; Todd J. Schwedt, Chia-Chun Chiang, Catherine D. Chong and David W. Dodick (2015), 'Functional MRI of migraine', *The Lancet Neurology*, 14 (1), pp.81–91, www.sciencedirect.com/science/article/abs/pii/S1474442214701930

2 Katarina Laurell, Ville Artto, Lars Bendtsen et al. (2016), 'Premonitory symptoms in migraine: A cross-sectional study in 2714 persons', *Cephalalgia*, 36 (10), pp.951–9, pubmed.ncbi.nlm.nih.gov/26643378; G. G. Schoonman, D. J. Evers, G. M. Terwindt et al. (2006), 'The prevalence of premonitory symptoms in migraine: A questionnaire study in 461 patients', *Cephalalgia,* 26 (10), pp.1209–13, pubmed.ncbi.nlm.nih.gov/16961788

3 Jean-Christophe Cuvellier (2019), 'Pediatric vs adult prodrome and postdrome: A window on migraine pathophysiology?', *Frontiers in Neurology*, 10, art.199, www.ncbi.nlm.nih.gov/pmc/articles/PMC6423905

4 International Headache Society (2018), 'Migraine without aura', International Classification of Headache Disorders, 3rd edn, ichd-3.org/1-migraine/1-1-migraine-without-aura

5 Michele Viana, Grazia Sances, Mattias Linde et al. (2017), 'Clinical features of migraine aura: Results from a prospective diary-aided study', *Cephalalgia*, 37 (10), pp.979–89, doi.org/10.1177/0333102416657147

6 Michele Viana, Erling Andreas Tronvik, Thien Phu Do et al. (2017), 'Clinical features of visual migraine aura: A systematic review and proposal of an official list', *Journal of Headache and Pain*, 20 (1), art.64, ihs-headache.org/wp-content/uploads/2020/06/3717_viana-poster-aura.pdf

7 Foxhall (2019), *Migraine: A History*

8 Viana, Tronvik, Phu Do et al. (2019), 'Clinical features of visual of migraine aura'

9 Katherine Foxhall (2016), 'Migraines were taken more seriously in medieval times – where did we go wrong?', University of Leicester Press Office, www2.le.ac.uk/offices/press/think-leicester/health-and-medicine/2016/

migraines-were-taken-more-seriously-in-medieval-times-2013-where-did-we-go-wrong

10 Cuvellier (2019), 'Pediatric vs adult prodrome and postdrome'

11 Ibid.

12 Elena C. Gross, Marco Lisicki, Dirk Fischer et al. (2019), 'The metabolic face of migraine – from pathophysiology to treatment', *Nature Reviews Neurology*, 15, pp.627–43, www.nature.com/articles/s41582-019-0255-4

13 Johns Hopkins Medicine (n.d.), 'How a migraine happens', https://www.hopkinsmedicine.org/health/conditions-and-diseases/headache/how-a-migraine-happens

14 Olga Cozzolino, Maria Marchese, Francesco Trovato et al. (2018), 'Understanding spreading depression from headache to sudden unexpected death', *Frontiers in Neurology*, 9, art.19, doi.org/10.3389/fneur.2018.00019; Andrew J. Whalen, Ying Xiao, Herve Kadji et al. (2018), 'Control of spreading depression with electrical fields', *Scientific Reports*, 8 (1), art.8769, www.nature.com/articles/s41598-018-26986-1

15 Yilong Cui, Yosky Kataoka and Yasuhoshi Watanabe (2014), 'Role of cortical spreading depression in the pathophysiology of migraine', *Neuroscience Bulletin*, 30 (5), pp.812–22, www.ncbi.nlm.nih.gov/pmc/articles/PMC5562594

16 For example, see Nazish Rafique, Lubna Ibrahim Al-Asoom, Rabia Latif et al. (2020), 'Prevalence of migraine and its relationship with psychological stress and sleep quality in female university students in Saudi Arabia', *Journal of Pain Research*, 13, pp.2423–30, pubmed.ncbi.nlm.nih.gov/33116786

17 Elizabeth Mostofsky, Suzanne M. Bertisch, Angeliki Vgontzas et al. (2020), 'Prospective cohort study of daily alcoholic beverage intake as a potential trigger of headaches among adults with episodic migraine', *Annals of Medicine*, 52 (7), pp.386–92, pubmed.ncbi.nlm.nih.gov/32306754

18 Hirohisa Okuma, Yumiko Okuma and Yasuhisa Kitagawa (2015), 'Examination of fluctuations in atmospheric pressure related to migraine', *SpringerPlus*, 4, art.790, www.ncbi.nlm.nih.gov/pmc/articles/PMC4684554; Hayrunnisa Bolay and Alan Rapoport (2011), 'Does low atmospheric pressure independently trigger migraine?', *Headache*, 51 (9), pp.1426–30, pubmed.ncbi.nlm.nih.gov/21906054

19 Kazuhito Kimoto, Saiko Aiba, Ryotaro Takashima et al. (2011), 'Influence of barometric pressure in patients with migraine headache', *Internal Medicine*, 50 (18), pp.1923–8, pubmed.ncbi.nlm.nih.gov/21921370

20 Jan Hoffmann and Ana Recober (2013), 'Migraine and triggers: Post hoc ergo propter hoc?', *Current Pain and Headache Reports*, 17 (10), art.370, www.ncbi.nlm.nih.gov/pmc/articles/PMC3857910

21 R. Salvesen and S. I. Bekkelund (2000), 'Migraine, as compared to other headaches, is worse during midnight-sun summer than during polar night: A questionnaire

study in an Arctic population', *Headache*, 40 (10), pp.824–9, pubmed.ncbi.nlm. nih.gov/11135027; Hallvard Lilleng and Srein Ivak Bekkelund (2010), 'Arctic environment triggers migraine attacks', *Canadian Family Physician*, 56 (6), pp. 549–51, www.ncbi.nlm.nih.gov/pmc/articles/PMC2902942

22 Paul R. Martin (2010), 'Behavioral management of migraine headache triggers: Learning to cope with triggers', *Current Pain and Headache Reports*, 14 (3), pp.221–7, pubmed.ncbi.nlm.nih.gov/20425190

3. When and What You Eat

1 Gökhan Evcili, Uygar Utku, Muhammed Nur Öğün and Gökhan Özdemir (2018), 'Early and long period follow-up results of low glycemic index diet for migraine prophylaxis', *Ağri*, 30 (1), pp.8–11, pubmed.ncbi.nlm.nih. gov/29450870

2 Innocenzo Rainero, Flora Govone, Annalisa Gai et al. (2018), 'Is migraine primarily a metaboloendocrine disorder?', *Current Pain and Headache Reports*, 22 (5), art.36, pubmed.ncbi.nlm.nih.gov/29619630; Claudia Bernecker, Sabine Pailer, Petra Kieslinger et al. (2010), 'GLP-2 and leptin are associated with hyperinsulinemia in non-obese female migraineurs', *Cephalagia*, 30 (11), pp. 1366–74, pubmed.ncbi.nlm.nih.gov/20959431; A. Fava, D. Pirritano, D. Consoli et al. (2014), 'Chronic migraine in women is associated with insulin resistance: A cross-sectional study', *European Journal of Neurology*, 21 (2), pp.267–72, pubmed. ncbi.nlm.nih.gov/24238370

3 These GI figures come from Weight Loss Resources, www.weightlossresources. co.uk/diet/gi_diet/glycaemic_index_tables.htm

4 Soodeh Razeghi Jahromi, Zeinab Ghorbani, Paolo Martelletti et al. (2019), 'Association of diet and headache', *Journal of Headache and Pain*, 20 (1), art.106, pubmed.ncbi.nlm.nih.gov/31726975

5 Wajeed Masoon, Pavan Annamaraju and Kalyan R. Uppaluri (2020), 'Ketogenic diet', *StatPearls*, www.ncbi.nlm.nih.gov/books/NBK499830; C. Di Lorenzo, G. Coppola, G. Sirianni et al. (2015), 'Migraine improvement during short lasting ketogenesis: A proof-of-concept study', *European Journal of Neurology*, 22 (1), pp.170–7, pubmed.ncbi.nlm.nih.gov/25156013

6 Marcelo E. Bigal, Richard B. Lipton, Philip R. Holland et al. (2007), 'Obesity, migraine, and chronic migraine: Possible mechanisms of interaction', *Neurology*, 68, pp.1851–61, www.drperlmutter.com/wp-content/uploads/2013/07/ 8-Obesity-migraine.pdf

7 Alberto Verrotti, Alessia Di Fonzo, Laura Penta et al. (2014), 'Obesity and headache/migraine: The importance of weight reduction through lifestyle modifications', *BioMed Research International*, 2014, www.ncbi.nlm.nih.gov/pmc/ articles/PMC3996319

8 Ruhan Karahan Özcan and Selen Gür Özmen (2019), 'The association between migraine, metabolic syndrome, insulin resistance, and obesity in women: A case-control study', *Şişli Etfal Hastanesi Tıp Bülteni*, 53 (4), pp.395–402, www.ncbi.nlm.nih.gov/pmc/articles/PMC7192290

9 Suresh Subramaniam and William A. Fletcher (2017), 'Obesity and weight loss in idiopathic intracranial hypertension: A narrative review', *Journal of Neuro-Ophthalmology*, 37 (2), pp.197–205, pubmed.ncbi.nlm.nih.gov/27636748

10 D. S. Bond, S. Vithiananthan, J. M. Nash et al. (2011), 'Improvement of migraine headaches in severely obese patients after bariatric surgery', *Neurology*, 76 (13), pp.1135–8, n.neurology.org/content/76/13/1135

11 Harvard Heart Letter (May 2009, updated 20 August 2019), 'No need to avoid healthy omega-6 fats', Harvard Medical School, www.health.harvard.edu/newsletter_article/no-need-to-avoid-healthy-omega-6-fats

12 Magdalena Nowaczewska, Michał Wiciński, Wojciech Kaźmierczak and Henryk Kaźmierczak (2020), 'To eat or not to eat: A review of the relationship between chocolate and migraines', *Nutrients*, 12 (3), art.608, www.ncbi.nlm.nih.gov/pmc/articles/PMC7146545

13 Elif Ilgaz Aydınlar, Pınar Yalınay Dikmen, Arzu Tiftikçi et al. (2013), 'IgG-based elimination diet in migraine plus irritable bowel syndrome', *Headache*, 53 (3), pp.514–25, pubmed.ncbi.nlm.nih.gov/23216231

14 F. Wantke, M. Götz and R. Jarisch (1993), 'Histamine-free diet: Treatment of choice for histamine-induced food intolerance and supporting treatment for chronic headaches', *Clinical & Experimental Allergy*, 23 (12), pp.982–5, pubmed.ncbi.nlm.nih.gov/10779289

15 Mahsa Arzani, Soodeh Razeghi Jahromi, Zeinab Ghorbani et al. (2020), 'Gut–brain axis and migraine headache: A comprehensive review', *Journal of Headache and Pain*, 21, thejournalofheadacheandpain.biomedcentral.com/articles/10.1186/s10194-020-1078-9

16 Melanie A. Heckman, Jorge Weil and Elvira Gonzalez de Mejia (2010), 'Caffeine (1, 3, 7-trimethylxanthine) in foods: A comprehensive review on consumption, functionality, safety, and regulatory matters', *Journal of Food Science*, 75 (3), pp.R77–87, doi.org/10.1111/j.1750-3841.2010.01561.x

17 Richard B. Lipton, Hans-Christoph Diener, Matthew S. Robbins et al. (2017), 'Caffeine in the management of patients with headache', *Journal of Headache and Pain*, 18 (1), art.107, www.ncbi.nlm.nih.gov/pmc/articles/PMC5655397

18 Gross, Lisicki, Fischer et al. (2019), 'The metabolic face of migraine – from pathophysiology to treatment'

19 Lisa A. Yablon and Alexander Mauskop (2011), 'Magnesium in headache', in R. Vink and M. Nechifor (eds), *Magnesium in the Central Nervous System* (Adelaide: University of Adelaide Press), www.ncbi.nlm.nih.gov/books/NBK507271

20 Başak Karakurum Göksel (2013), 'The use of complementary and alternative medicine in patients with migraine', *Nöropsikiyatri Arşsivi*, 50 (Suppl. 7), pp.S41–6, www.ncbi.nlm.nih.gov/pmc/articles/PMC5353077

21 Gross, Lisicki, Fischer et al. (2019), 'The metabolic face of migraine – from pathophysiology to treatment'

22 Tae-Jin Song, Min-Kyung Chu, Jong-Hee Sohn et al. (2018), 'Effect of vitamin D deficiency on the frequency of headaches in migraine', *Journal of Clinical Neurology*, 14 (3), pp.366–73, www.ncbi.nlm.nih.gov/pmc/articles/PMC6031995

23 Marilia Carabotti, Annunziata Scirocco, Maria Antonietta Maselli and Carola Severi (2015), 'The gut–brain axis: Interactions between enteric microbiota, central and enteric nervous systems', *Annals of Gastroenterology*, 28 (2), pp.203–9, www.ncbi.nlm.nih.gov/pmc/articles/PMC4367209

24 Arşani, Jahromi, Ghorbani et al. (2020), 'Gut–brain axis and migraine headache'

4. Exercising Body and Brain

1 E. Köseoglu, A. Akboyraz, A. Soyuer et al. (2003), 'Aerobic exercise and plasma beta endorphin levels in patients with migrainous headache without aura', *Cephalalgia*, 23 (10), pp.972–6, pubmed.ncbi.nlm.nih.gov/14984230

2 Rosaria Greco, Valeria Gasperi, Mauro Maccarrone and Cristina Tassorelli (2010), 'The endocannabinoid system and migraine', *Experimental Neurology*, 22 (1), pp.85–91, pubmed.ncbi.nlm.nib.gov/20353780

3 A. Deitrich and W. F. McDaniel (2004), 'Endocannabinoids and exercise', *British Journal of Sports Medicine*, 38 (5), pp.536–41, bjsm.bmj.com/content/38/5/536

4 Faisal Mohammad Amin, Stavroula Aristeidou, Carlo Baraldi et al. (2018), 'The association between migraine and physical exercise', *Journal of Headache and Pain*, 19, art.83, www.ncbi.nlm.nih.gov/pmc/articles/PMC6134860

5 Emma Varkey, Åsa Cider, Jane Carlsson et al. (2011), 'Exercise as migraine prophylaxis: A randomized study using relaxation and topiramate as controls', *Cephalalgia*, 31 (14), pp.1428–38, journals.sagepub.com/doi/10.1177/0333102411419681

6 Claudia H. Overath, Stephanie Darabaneanu, Marie C. Evers et al. (2014), 'Does an aerobic endurance programme have an influence on information processing in migraineurs?', *Journal of Headache and Pain*, 15 (1), art.11, www.ncbi.nlm.nih.gov/pmc/articles/PMC4017768

7 UK Chief Medical Officer (2019), Physical activity guidelines 2019, assets.publishing.service.gov.uk/government/uploads/system/uploads/attachment_data/file/829884/3-physical-activity-for-adults-and-older-adults.pdf

8 Amin, Aristeidou, Baraldi et al. (2018), 'The association between migraine and physical exercise'

9 Ibid.

10 Cantor Tarperi, Fabian Sanchis-Gomar, Martina Montagnana et al. (2020), 'Effects of endurance exercise on serum concentration of calcitonin gene-related peptide (CGRP): A potential link between exercise intensity and headache', *Clinical Chemistry and Laboratory Medicine*, 58 (10), pp.1707–12, doi. org/10.1515/cclm-2019-1337

11 Ravikiran Kisan, M. U. Sujan, Meghana Adoor et al. (2014), 'Effect of yoga on migraine: A comprehensive study using clinical profile and cardiac autonomic functions', *International Journal of Yoga*, 7 (2), pp.126–32, www.ncbi.nlm.nih.gov/pmc/articles/PMC4097897

12 Ryan B. Abbott, Ka-Kit Hui, Ron D. Hays et al. (2007), 'A randomized controlled trial of tai chi for tension headaches', *Evidence-based Complementary and Alternative Medicine*, 4 (1), pp.107–13, www.ncbi.nlm.nih.gov/pmc/articles/PMC1810369

13 Yao Jie Xie, Stanley Sai-chuen Hui, Suzanne C. Ho et al. (2018), 'The effectiveness of 12-week tai chi training on the migraine attack days, body composition, and blood pressure in Chinese women with episodic migraine: A randomized controlled trial', *Circulation*, 137, Abstract P034, www.ahajournals.org/doi/10.1161/circ.137.suppl_1.p034

14 Adam S. Sprouse-Blum, Alexandra K. Gabriel, Jon P. Brown and Melvin H. C. Yee (2013), 'Randomized controlled trial: Targeted neck cooling in the treatment of the migraine patient', *Hawai'i Journal of Medicine & Public Health*, 72 (7), pp. 237–41, www.ncbi.nlm.nih.gov/pmc/articles/PMC3727573

15 Serap Ucler, Ozlem Coskun, Levent E. Inan and Yonca Kanatli (2006), 'Cold therapy in migraine patients: Open-label, non-controlled, pilot study', *Evidence-based Complementary and Alternative Medicine*, 3 (4), pp.489–93, www.ncbi.nlm.nih. gov/pmc/articles/PMC1697736

16 Anon. (7 April 2019), 'Migraine sufferer completes 100-day cold-water challenge', BBC News, www.bbc.co.uk/news/uk-wales-47831576; '100 Days of Vitamin Sea', www.vitaminseafilm.com

17 M. J. Tipton, N. Collier, H. Massey et al. (2017), 'Cold water immersion: Kill or cure?', *Experimental Physiology*, 102 (11), pp.1335–55, doi.org/10.1113/EP086283

18 Jeppe Hvedstrup, Lærke Tørring Kolding, Messoud Ashina et al. (2020), 'Increased neck muscle stiffness in migraine patients with ictal neck pain: A shear wave elastography study', *Cephalalgia*, 40 (6), pp.565–74, doi. org/10.1177/0333102420919998

19 Gabriela F. Carvalho, Kerstin Luedtke, Tibor M. Szikszay et al. (2020), 'Muscle endurance training of the neck triggers migraine attacks', *Cephalalgia*, online first (17 November 2020), doi.org/10.1177/0333102420970184

20 Sun-Myung Lee, Chang-Hyung Lee, David O'Sullivan, Joo-Ha Jung and Jung-Jun Park (2016), 'Clinical effectiveness of a Pilates treatment for forward head

posture', *Journal of Physical Therapy Science*, 28 (7), pp.2009–13, www.ncbi.nlm.nih.gov/pmc/articles/PMC4968495/

5. Getting Better Sleep

1 Yu-Kai Lin, Guan-Yu Lin, Jiunn-Tay Lee et al. (2016), 'Associations between sleep quality and migraine frequency: A cross-sectional case-control study', *Medicine*, 95 (17), e3554, www.ncbi.nlm.nih.gov/pmc/articles/PMC4998727

2 Leslie Kelman and Jeanetta C. Rains (2005), 'Headache and sleep: Examination of sleep patterns and complaints in a large clinical sample of migraineurs', *Headache*, 45 (7), pp.904–10, pubmed.ncbi.nlm.nih.gov/15985108

3 Jean-Philippe Chaput, Caroline Dutil and Hugues Sampasa-Kanyinga (2018), 'Sleeping hours: What is the ideal number and how does age impact this?', *Nature and Science of Sleep*, 10, pp.421–30, www.ncbi.nlm.nih.gov/pmc/articles/PMC6267703

4 Marcelo R. Masruha, Jaime Lin, Domingo S. de Souza Vieira et al. (2010), 'Urinary 6-sulphatoxymelatonin levels are depressed in chronic migraine and several comorbidities', *Headache*, 50 (3), pp.413–19, pubmed.ncbi.nlm.nih.gov/19817880

5 Harvard Mental Health Letter (2019), 'Sleep and mental health', Harvard Medical School www.health.harvard.edu/newsletter_article/Sleep-and-mental-health

6 Ping-Kun Chen, Jong-Ling Fuh, Hsien-Yuan Lane et al. (2011), 'Morning headache in habitual snorers: Frequency, characteristics, predictors and impacts', *Cephalalgia*, 31 (7), pp.829–36, pubmed.ncbi.nlm.nih.gov/21602422

7 Keisuke Suzuki, Masayuki Miyamoto, Tomoyuki Mikamoto et al. (2015), 'Sleep apnoea headache in obstructive sleep apnoea syndrome patients presenting with morning headache: Comparison of the ICHD-2 and ICHD-3 beta criteria', *Journal of Headache and Pain*, 16, art.56, www.ncbi.nlm.nih.gov/pmc/articles/PMC4478186

8 Marina Ruiz, Patricia Mulero, María Isabel Pedraza et al. (2015), 'From wakefulness to sleep: Migraine and hypnic headache association in a series of 23 patients', *Headache*, 55 (1), pp.167–73, pubmed.ncbi.nlm.nih.gov/25319633

9 Dagny Holle and Mark Obermann (2012), 'Hypnic headache and caffeine', *Expert Review of Neurotherapeutics*, 12 (9), pp.1125–32, pubmed.ncbi.nlm.nih.gov/23039391

6. Managing Your Mental Health

1 Cecilia Camarda, Carmela Pipia, Antonia Taglialavori et al. (2008), 'Comorbidity between depressive symptoms and migraine: Preliminary data from the Zabút

Aging Project', *Neurological Sciences*, 29 (Suppl. 1), pp. S149–51, pubmed.ncbi.nlm.nih.gov/18545919

2 Qiang Gu, Jin-Chao Hou and Xiang-Ming Fang (2018), 'Mindfulness meditation for primary headache pain: A meta-analysis', *Chinese Medical Journal*, 131 (7), pp.829–38, www.ncbi.nlm.nih.gov/pmc/articles/PMC5887742

3 Amy B. Wachholtz, Christopher D. Malone and Kenneth I. Pargament (2017), 'Effect of different meditation types on migraine headache medication use', *Behavioral Medicine*, 43 (1), pp.1–8, pubmed.ncbi.nlm.nih.gov/25864906

4 Pamela J. D'Souza, Mark A. Lumley, Christina A. Kraft and John A. Dooley (2008), 'Relaxation training and written emotional disclosure for tension or migraine headaches: A randomized, controlled trial', *Annals of Behavioral Medicine*, 36 (1), pp.21–32, www.ncbi.nlm.nih.gov/pmc/articles/PMC2931412; Andrea N. Niles, Kate E. Byrne Haltom, Catherine M. Mulvenna et al. (2014), 'Effects of expressive writing on psychological and physical& health: The moderating role of emotional expressivity', *Anxiety, Stress, & Coping*, 27 (1), pp.1–17, www.ncbi.nlm.nih.gov/pmc/articles/PMC3830620

5 Randy A. Sansone and Lori A. Sansone (2010), 'Gratitude and wellbeing', *Psychiatry*, 7 (11), pp.18–22, www.ncbi.nlm.nih.gov/pmc/articles/PMC3010965; D. E. Davis, E. Choe, J. Meyers et al. (2016), 'Thankful for the little things: A meta-analysis of gratitude interventions', *Journal of Counseling Psychology*, 63 (1), pp.20–31, doi.org/10.1037/cou0000107

6 Niamh Flynn (2018), 'Systematic review of the effectiveness of hypnosis for the management of headache', *International Journal of Clinical and Experimental Hypnosis*, 66 (4), pp.343–52, pubmed.ncbi.nlm.nih.gov/30152733

7 Valentine Seymour (2016), 'The human–nature relationship and its impact on health: A critical review', *Frontiers in Public Health*, 4, art.260, pubmed.ncbi.nlm.nih.gov/27917378; David G. Pearson and Tony Craig (2014), 'The great outdoors?: Exploring the mental health benefits of natural environments', *Frontiers in Psychology*, 5, art.1178, doi.org/10.3389/fpsyg.2014.01178; Lisa Wood, Paula Hooper, Sarah Foster and Fiona Bull (2017), 'Public green spaces and positive mental health: Investigating the relationship between access, quantity and types of parks and mental wellbeing', *Health & Place*, 48, pp.63–71, doi.org/10.1016/j.healthplace.2017.09.002

8 Todd A. Smitherman and Steven M. Baskin (2016), 'Depression and anxiety in migraine patients', American Migraine Foundation, americanmigrainefoundation.org/resource-library/anxiety-and-depression

9 Ibid.

10 Birk Engmann (2012), 'Bipolar affective disorder and migraine', *Case Reports in Medicine*, 2012, art.389851, www.ncbi.nlm.nih.gov/pmc/articles/PMC3357514

11 Gretchen E. Tietjen and B. Lee Peterlin (2011), 'Childhood abuse and migraine: Epidemiology, sex differences, and potential mechanisms', *Headache*, 51 (6), pp. 869–79, www.ncbi.nlm.nih.gov/pmc/articles/PMC3972492

12 E. A. MacGregor, J. Brandes, A. Eikermann and R. Giammarco (2004), 'Impact of migraine on patients and their families: The Migraine And Zolmitriptan Evaluation (MAZE) survey – phase III', *Current Medical Research and Opinion*, 20 (7), pp.1143–50, pubmed.ncbi.nlm.nih.gov/15265259

13 Richard B. Lipton, Dawn C. Buse, Aubrey Manack Adams et al. (2017), 'Family impact of migraine: Development of the Impact of Migraine on Partners and Adolescent Children (IMPAC) Scale', *Headache*, 57 (4), pp.570–85, www.ncbi.nlm.nih.gov/pmc/articles/PMC5396278

14 Amanda L. Hall, Dina Karvounides, Amy A. Gelfand et al. (2019), 'Improving the patient experience with Migraine Camp, a one-day group intervention for adolescents with chronic headache and their parents', *Headache*, 59 (8), pp.1392–1400, www.ncbi.nlm.nih.gov/pmc/articles/PMC7316641

7. Rescue Plans for Acute Attacks

1 Miguel J. A. Láinez, Ana García-Casado and Francisco Gascón (2013), 'Optimal management of severe nausea and vomiting in migraine: Improving patient outcomes', *Patient Related Outcome Measures*, 4, pp.61–73, www.ncbi.nlm.nih.gov/pmc/articles/PMC3798203

2 Sheena Derry and R. Andrew Moore (2013), 'Paracetamol (acetaminophen) with or without an antiemetic for acute migraine headaches in adults', *Cochrane Database of Systematic Reviews*, 2013 (4), art.CD008040, pubmed.ncbi.nlm.nih.gov/23633349

3 The Medical Letter (2017), 'The Medical Letter on drugs and therapeutics: Triptans', www.headache.mobi/uploads/1/1/7/5/11757140/triptans.pdf

4 NICE (2018), 'Migraine', bnf.nice.org.uk/treatment-summary/migraine.html

8. Migraine Preventers

1 Rujin Long, Yousheng Zhu and Shusheng Zhou (2019), 'Therapeutic role of melatonin in migraine prophylaxis: A systematic review', *Medicine*, 98 (3), e14099, www.ncbi.nlm.nih.gov/pmc/articles/PMC6370052

2 Lin Han, Yao Liu, Hai Xiong and Peiwei Hong (2019), 'CGRP monoclonal antibody for preventive treatment of chronic migraine: An update of meta-analysis', *Brain and Behavior*, 9 (2), e01215, www.ncbi.nlm.nih.gov/pmc/articles/PMC6379644

3 James E. Frampton and Stephen Silberstein (2018), 'OnabotulinumtoxinA: A review in the prevention of chronic migraine', *Drugs*, 78 (5), pp.589–600, www.ncbi.nlm.nih.gov/pmc/articles/PMC5915521

4 Olivia Begasse de Dhaem, Mohammad Hadi Gharedaghi and Paul Rizzoli (2020), 'Modifications to the PREEMPT protocol for OnabotulinumtoxinA

injections for chronic migraine in clinical practice', *Headache*, 60 (7), pp.1365–75, pubmed.ncbi.nlm.nih.gov/32335918

5   K. Linde, G. Allais, B. Brinkhaus et al. (2016), 'Acupuncture for preventing migraine attacks', *Cochrane Database of Systematic Reviews*, 2016 (6), art.CD001218, www.cochrane.org/CD001218/SYMPT_acupuncture-preventing-migraine-attacks

6   British Acupuncture Council (n.d.), 'Migraine and acupuncture: The evidence for effectiveness', www.acupuncture.org.uk/a-to-z-of-conditions/public-review-papers/378-migraine-and-acupuncture-the-evidence-for-effectiveness.html

7   American Migraine Foundation (2017), 'Daith piercings & migraines', americanmigrainefoundation.org/resource-library/daith-piercings-101

8   Migraine Buddy (2018), 'Daith piercings x migraines', migrainebuddy.com/blog/2018/9/17/daith-piercings-x-migraine-buddy

9   Sonja Vučković, Dragana Srebro, Katarina Savić Vujović et al. (2018), 'Cannabinoids and pain: New insights from old molecules', *Frontiers in Pharmacology*, 9, art.1259, pubmed.ncbi.nlm.nih.gov/30542280

10 Foxhall (2019), *Migraine: A History*

11 Eric P. Baron, Philippe Lucas, Joshua Eades and Olivia Hogue (2018), 'Patterns of medicinal cannabis use, strain analysis, and substitution effect among patients with migraine, headache, arthritis, and chronic pain in a medicinal cannabis cohort', *Journal of Headache and Pain*, 19 (1), art.37, pubmed.ncbi.nlm.nih.gov/29797104

12 Healthwise Staff (2019), 'Stress management: Doing progressive muscle relaxation', University of Michigan Medical School, www.uofmhealth.org/health-library/uz2225

13 Gay L. Lipchik (2016), 'Biofeedback and relaxation training for headaches', American Migraine Foundation, americanmigrainefoundation.org/resource-library/biofeedback-and-relaxation-training

14 Francesco Cerritelli, Eleonora Lacorte, Nuria Ruffini and Nicola Vanacore (14 March 2017), 'Osteopathy for primary headache patients: A systematic review', *Journal of Pain Research*, 10, pp.601–11, www.ncbi.nlm.nih.gov/pmc/articles/PMC5359118

9. Women and Hormones

1   Jelena M. Pavlović, Amanda A. Allshouse, Nanette F. Santoro et al. (2016), 'Sex hormones in women with and without migraine', *Neurology*, 87 (1), pp.49–56, www.ncbi.nlm.nih.gov/pmc/articles/PMC4932235

2   Gretchen E. Tietjen, Anita Conway, Christine Utley et al. (2006), 'Migraine is associated with menorrhagia and endometriosis', *Headache*, 46 (3), pp.422–8, pubmed.ncbi.nlm.nih.gov/16618258

3   Pavlović, Allshouse, Santoro et al. (2016), 'Sex hormones in women with and without migraine'

4 Jelena Pavlović (2020), 'The impact of midlife on migraine in women: Summary of current views', *Women's Midlife Health*, 6, art.11, www.ncbi.nlm.nih.gov/pmc/articles/PMC7542111; Patrizia Ripa, Raffaele Ornello, Diana Degan et al. (2015), 'Migraine in menopausal women: A systematic review', *International Journal of Women's Health*, 7, pp.773–82, www.ncbi.nlm.nih.gov/pmc/articles/PMC4548761; Vincent T. Martin, Jelena Pavlović, Kristina M. Fanning et al. (2016), 'Perimenopause and menopause are associated with high frequency headache in women with migraine: Results of the American Migraine Prevalence and Prevention Study', *Headache*, 56 (2), pp.292–305, pubmed.ncbi.nlm.nih.gov/26797693

5 Alejandro Labastida-Ramírez, Eloísa Rubio-Beltrán, Carlos M. Villalón and Antoinette Maassen Van Den Brink (2019), 'Gender aspects of CGRP in migraine', *Cephalalgia*, 39 (3), pp.435–44, www.ncbi.nlm.nih.gov/pmc/articles/PMC6402050; Zoë Delaruelle, Tatiana A. Ivanova, Sabrina Khan et al. (2018), 'Male and female sex hormones in primary headaches', *Journal of Headache and Pain*, 19, art.117, doi.org/10.1186/s10194-018-0922-7

6 ICHD-3 (2018), 'Pure menstrual migraine without aura', ichd-3.org/appendix/a1-migraine/a1-1-migraine-without-aura/a1-1-1-pure-menstrual-migraine-without-aura

7 Elizabeth Sullivan and Cheryl Bushnell (2010), 'Management of menstrual migraine: A review of current abortive and prophylactic therapies', *Current Pain and Headache Reports*, 14 (5), pp.376–84, www.ncbi.nlm.nih.gov/pmc/articles/PMC2989388; Anne H. Calhoun (2012), 'Menstrual migraine: Update on pathophysiology and approach to therapy and management', *Current Treatment Options in Neurology*, 14 (1), pp.1–14, pubmed.ncbi.nlm.nih.gov/22072055

8 Andrea G. Edlow and Deborah Bartz (2010), 'Hormonal contraceptive options for women with headache: A review of evidence', *Obstetrics & Gynecology*, 3 (2), pp.55–65, www.ncbi.nlm.nih.gov/pmc/articles/PMC2938905

9 Chrisandra L. Shufelt and C. Noel Bairey Merz (2009), 'Contraceptive hormone use and cardiovascular disease', *Journal of the American College of Cardiology*, 53 (3), pp.221–31, www.ncbi.nlm.nih.gov/pmc/articles/PMC2660203

10 'Valproate pregnancy-prevention programme: Actions required now from GPs, specialists, and dispensers' (2018), www.gov.uk/drug-safety-update/valproate-pregnancy-prevention-programme-actions-required-now-from-gps-specialists-and-dispensers

11 Waldmiro Antônio Diégues Serva, Vilneide Maria Santos Braga Diégues Serva, Maria de Fátima Costa Caminha et al. (2011), 'Course of migraine during pregnancy among migraine sufferers before pregnancy', *Arquivos de neuro-psiquiatria*, 69 (4), pp.613–19, pubmed.ncbi.nlm.nih.gov/21877029

12 A. Negro, Z. Delaruelle, T. A. Ivanova et al. (2017), 'Headache and pregnancy: A systematic review', *Journal of Headache and Pain*, 18 (1), art.106, www.ncbi.nlm.nih.gov/pmc/articles/PMC5648730

13 G. Sances, F. Granella, R. E. Nappi et al. (2003), 'Course of migraine during pregnancy and postpartum: A prospective study', *Cephalalgia*, 23 (3), pp.197–205, doi.org/10.1046/j.1468-2982.2003.00480.x

14 Archana Dixit, Manish Bhardwaj and Bhavna Sharma (2012), 'Headache in pregnancy: A nuisance or a new sense?', *Obstetrics and Gynecology International*, 2012, art.697697, www.ncbi.nlm.nih.gov/pmc/articles/PMC3306951

15 Best Use of Medicines in Pregnancy (bumps), www.medicinesinpregnancy.org/Medicine--pregnancy

16 Todd J. Schwedt, Kathleen Digre, Stewart J. Tepper et al. (2020), 'The American Registry for Migraine Research: Research methods and baseline data for an initial patient cohort', *Headache*, 60 (2), pp.337–47, pubmed.ncbi.nlm.nih.gov/31755111; Thomas Folkmann Hansen, Mona Ameri Chalmer, Thilde Marie Haspang et al. (2019), 'Predicting treatment response using pharmacy register in migraine', *Journal of Headache and Pain*, 20, art.31, doi.org/10.1186/s10194-019-0987-y; Silvia Duong, Pina Bozzo, Hedvig Nordeng and Adrienne Einarson (2010), 'Safety of triptans for migraine headaches during pregnancy and breast-feeding', *Canadian Family Physician*, 56 (6), pp.537–9, www.ncbi.nlm.nih.gov/pmc/articles/PMC2902939

17 Siri Amundsen, Hedvig Nordeng, Ole-Martin Fuskevåg et al. (2019), 'Transfer of triptans into human breast milk and estimation of infant drug exposure through breastfeeding', *Reproductive Toxicology*, 88, p.141, doi.org/10.1016/j.reprotox.2019.05.032

18 Duong, Bozzo, Nordeng and Einarson (2010), 'Safety of triptans for migraine headaches during pregnancy and breastfeeding'

19 National Library of Medicine, Drugs and Lactation Database (LactMed), www.ncbi.nlm.nih.gov/books/NBK501922

20 Breastfeeding Network, www.breastfeedingnetwork.org.uk/migraines

21 Shazia K. Afridi (2018), 'Current concepts in migraine and their relevance to pregnancy', *Obstetric Medicine*, 11 (4), pp.154–9, www.ncbi.nlm.nih.gov/pmc/articles/PMC6295770

22 Gad Rennert, Hedy S. Rennert, Mila Pinchev et al. (2009), 'Use of hormone replacement therapy and the risk of colorectal cancer', *Journal of Clinical Oncology*, 27 (27), pp.4542–7, www.ncbi.nlm.nih.gov/pmc/articles/PMC2754905; Edoardo Botteri, Nathalie C. Støer, Solveig Sakshaug et al. (2017), 'Menopausal hormone therapy and colorectal cancer: A linkage between nationwide registries in Norway', *BMJ Open*, 7 (11), e017639, bmjopen.bmj.com/content/7/11/e017639

23 Bo von Schoultz (2009), 'Oestrogen therapy: Oral versus non-oral administration', *Gynecological Endocrinology*, 25 (9), pp.551–3, doi.org/10.1080/09513590902836551

24 Rebecca Glaser, Constantine Dimitrakakis, Nancy Trimble and Vincent Martin (2012), 'Testosterone pellet implants and migraine headaches: A pilot study', *Maturitas*, 71 (4), pp.385–8, pubmed.ncbi.nlm.nih.gov/22310106

25 British Menopause Society, 'Migraine and HRT', thebms.org.uk/publications/
    tools-for-clinicians/migraine-and-hrt

26 E. Anne MacGregor and Antoinette Maassen van den Brink (2019), 'Trans-
    gender and migraine', in *Gender and Migraine* (Springer ebook), pp.113–27, link.
    springer.com/chapter/10.1007/978-3-030-02988-3_9

27 Anna Maria Aloisi, Valeria Bachiocco, Antonietta Costantino et al. (2007),
    'Cross-sex hormone administration changes pain in transsexual women and
    men', *Pain*, 132 (Suppl.1), pp.S60–7, pubmed.ncbi.nlm.nih.gov/17379410

10. Children with Migraine

1   Heather Angus-Leppan, Defne Saatci, Alastair Sutcliffe and Roberto J. Guiloff
    (2018), 'Abdominal Migraine', *BMJ*, 360, art.k179, pubmed.ncbi.nlm.nih.
    gov/29459383/

2   N. Karsan, P. Prabhakar and P. J. Goadsby (2016), 'Characterising the premoni-
    tory stage of migraine in children: A clinic-based study of 100 patients in a
    specialist headache service', *Journal of Headache and Pain*, 17 (1), art.94, www.
    ncbi.nlm.nih.gov/pmc/articles/PMC5074936

3   Raluca Ioana Teleanu et al. (2016), 'Treatment of pediatric migraine: A review',
    Mædica, 11 (2), pp.136–43, www.ncbi.nlm.nih.gov/pmc/articles/PMC5394581

4   David Kernick, Deborah Reinhold and John L. Campbell (2009), 'Impact of
    headache on young people in a school population', *British Journal of General Prac-
    tice*, 59 (566), pp.678–81, www.ncbi.nlm.nih.gov/pmc/articles/PMC2734356

5   P. Fearon and M. Hotopf (2001), 'Relation between headache in childhood and
    physical and psychiatric symptoms in adulthood: National birth cohort study',
    BMJ, 322 (7295), art.1145, pubmed.ncbi.nlm.nih.gov/11348907

6   H. G. Farquhar (1956), 'Abdominal migraine in children', *BMJ* (7), 4975, p.1082,
    www.bmj.com/content/1/4975/1082

7   Irene Patniyot and William Qubty (2020), 'Short-term treatment of migraine in
    children and adolescents', *JAMA Pediatrics*, 174 (8), pp.789–90, pubmed.ncbi.
    nlm.nih.gov/32568383

8   A. D. Hershey, S. W. Powers, A.-L. B. Vockell et al. (2004), 'Development of
    a patient-based grading scale for PedMIDAS', *Cephalalgia*, 24 (10), pp.844–9,
    journals.sagepub.com/doi/full/10.1111/j.1468-2982.2004.00757.x; Children's
    Hospital Medical Center (2001), 'PhenX toolkit (data collection worksheet),
    www.phenxtoolkit.org/toolkit_content/PDF/PX130502.pdf

9   Tietjen, Conway, Utley et al. (2006), 'Migraine is associated with menorrhagia
    and endometriosis'

10 Noemi Faedda, Rita Cerutti, Paola Verdecchia et al. (2016), 'Behavioral manage-
    ment of headache in children and adolescents', *Journal of Headache and Pain*, 17
    (1), art.80, pubmed.ncbi.nlm.nih.gov/27596923

11 Ibid.

12 Lawrence Richer, Lori Billinghurst, Meghan A. Linsdell et al. (2016), 'Drugs for the acute treatment of migraine in children and adolescents', *Cochrane Database of Systematic Reviews*, 2016 (4), art.CD005220, doi.org/10.1002/14651858. CD005220.pub2

13 Maryam Oskoui, Tamara Pringsheim, Lori Billinghurst et al. (2019), 'Practice guideline update summary: Pharmacologic treatment for pediatric migraine prevention', *Neurology*, 93 (11), pp.500–9, doi.org/10.1212/WNL.0000000000008105

14 Teleanu et al. (2016), 'Treatment of pediatric migraine: A review'

15 Seyed Hassan Tonekaboni, Ahad Ghazavi, Afshin Fayyazi et al. (2013), 'Prophylaxis of childhood migraine: Topiromate versus propranolol', *Iranian Journal of Child Neurology*, 7 (1), pp.9–14, www.ncbi.nlm.nih.gov/pmc/articles/ PMC3943076

16 Scott W. Powers, Christopher S. Coffey, Leigh A. Chamberlin et al. (2017), 'Trial of amitriptyline, topiramate, and placebo for pediatric migraine', *New England Journal of Medicine*, 376 (2), pp.115–24, www.nejm.org/doi/full/10.1056/ NEJMoa1610384

17 Joanne Kacperski, Antoinette Green and Sharoon Qaiser (2020), 'Management of chronic migraine in children and adolescents: A brief discussion on preventive therapies', *Paediatric Drugs*, 22 (6), pp.635–43, pubmed.ncbi.nlm.nih. gov/32889686

18 Nick Peter Barnes and Elizabeth Katherine James (2009), 'Migraine headache in children', *BMJ Clinical Evidence*, 2009, art.0318, www.ncbi.nlm.nih.gov/pmc/ articles/PMC2907773

19 Man Amanat, Mansoureh Togha, Elmira Agah et al. (2019), 'Cinnarizine and sodium valproate as the preventive agents of pediatric migraine: A randomized double-blind placebo-controlled trial', *Cephalalgia*, 40 (7), pp.665–74, doi. org/10.1177/0333102419888485

20 'Valproate pregnancy-prevention programme: Actions required now from GPs, specialists, and dispensers' (2018)

21 Razieh Fallah, Fatemeh Fazelishoroki and Leila Sekhavat (2018), 'A randomized clinical trial comparing the efficacy of melatonin and amitriptyline in migraine prophylaxis of children', *Iranian Journal of Child Neurology*, 12 (1), pp.47–54, www. ncbi.nlm.nih.gov/pmc/articles/PMC5760673

22 Paul K. Winner, Marielle Kabbouce, Marcy Yonker et al., (2020), 'A randomized trial to evaluate OnabotulinumtoxinA for prevention of headaches in adolescents with chronic migraine', *Headache*, 60 (3), pp.564–75, www.ncbi.nlm.nih. gov/pmc/articles/PMC7065250; Marielle Kabbouche, Hope O'Brien and Andrew D. Hershey (2012), 'OnabotulinumtoxinA in pediatric chronic daily headache', *Current Neurology and Neuroscience Reports*, 12 (2), pp.114–17, pubmed.ncbi.nlm.nih.gov/22274570; Valerie W. Chan, E. Jane McCabe and Daune

L. MacGregor (2009), 'Botox treatment for migraine and chronic daily headache in adolescents', *Journal of Neuroscience Nursing*, 41 (5), pp.235–43, pubmed.ncbi.nlm.nih.gov/19835236

23 Kernick, Reinhold and Campbell (2009), 'Impact of headache on young people in a school population'

11. Working with Migraine

1 United Nations, 'Disability Laws and Acts by Country/Area', www.un.org/development/desa/disabilities/disability-laws-and-acts-by-country-area.html

2 Work Foundation (2018), 'Society's headache: The socioeconomic impact of migraine', www.lancaster.ac.uk/media/lancaster-university/content-assets/documents/lums/work-foundation/SocietysHeadacheTheSocioeconomicimpactofmigraine.pdf

3 US Department of Health and Human Services (2020), 'Estimates of funding for various research, condition, and disease categories', 24 February 2020, report.nih.gov/categorical_spending.aspx

4 European Migraine & Headache Alliance (2020), 'Migraine at work', www.emhalliance.org/wp-content/uploads/2020/01/EMHA-Migraine-at-work.pdf

12. Migraine Variants

1 International Headache Society (2018), International Classification of Headache Disorders, 3rd edn [ICHD-3], ichd-3.org

2 Marianne Deiterich, Mark Obermann and Nese Celebisoy (2016), 'Vestibular migraine: The most frequent entity of episodic vertigo', *Journal of Neurology*, 263, pp.82–9, www.ncbi.nlm.nih.gov/pmc/articles/PMC4833782

3 Thomas Lempert, Jes Olesen, Joseph Furman et al. (2012), 'Vestibular migraine: Diagnostic criteria', *Journal of Vestibular Research*, 22 (4), pp.167–72, pubmed.ncbi.nlm.nih.gov/23142830

4 ICHD-3 (2018), 'Vestibular migraine', ichd-3.org/appendix/a1-migraine/a1-6-episodic-syndromes-that-may-be-associated-with-migraine/a1-6-6-vestibular-migraine

5 Anthony A. Mikulec, Farhoud Faraji and Laurence J. Kinsella (2012), 'Evaluation of the efficacy of caffeine cessation, nortriptyline, and topiramate therapy in vestibular migraine and complex dizziness of unknown etiology', *American Journal of Otolaryngology*, 33 (1), pp.121–7, pubmed.ncbi.nlm.nih.gov/21704423

6 Jessica Vitkovic, Arimbi Winoto, Gary Rance et al. (2013), 'Vestibular rehabilitation outcomes in patients with and without vestibular migraine', *Journal of Neurology*, 260 (12), pp.3039–48, pubmed.ncbi.nlm.nih.gov/24061769

7 ICHD-3 (2018), 'Hemiplegic migraine', ichd-3.org/1-migraine/1-2-migraine-with-aura/1-2-3-hemiplegic-migraine

8 Anil Kumar, Debopam Samanta, Prabhu D. Emmady and Rohan Arora (2020), 'Hemiplegic migraine', *StatPearls*, www.ncbi.nlm.nih.gov/books/NBK513302

9 Yasir Al Khalili, Sameer Jain and Kevin C. King (2020), 'Retinal migraine headache', *StatPearls*, www.ncbi.nlm.nih.gov/books/NBK507725

10 ICHD-3 (2018), 'Typical aura without headache', ichd-3.org/1-migraine/1-2-migraine-with-aura/1-2-1-migraine-with-typical-aura/1-2-1-2-typical-aura-without-headache

11 ICHD-3 (2018), 'Migraine with brainstem aura', ichd-3.org/1-migraine/1-2-migraine-with-aura/1-2-2-migraine-with-brainstem-aura

12 The Migraine Trust (2020), 'Migraine with brainstem aura', www.migrainetrust.org/about-migraine/types-of-migraine/migraine-with-brainstem-aura

13 Geneviève Dermarquay, Anne Ducros, Alexandra Montavont et al. (2018), 'Migraine with brainstem aura: Why not a cortical origin?', *Cephalalgia*, 38 (10), pp.1687–95, journals.sagepub.com/doi/full/10.1177/0333102417738251

13. Cluster and Other Headaches

1 International Headache Society (2018), 'Other primary headache disorders', International Classification of Headache Disorders, 3rd edn [ICHD-3], ichd-3.org/other-primary-headache-disorders

2 Paola Torelli and Gian Camillo Manzoni (2005), 'Behavior during cluster headache', *Current Pain and Headache Reports*, 9 (2), pp.113–19, pubmed.ncbi.nlm.nih.gov/15745621

3 Alina Buture, Fayyaz Ahmed, Lisa Dikomitis and Jason W. Boland (2019), 'Systematic literature review on the delays in the diagnosis and misdiagnosis of cluster headache', *Neurological Sciences*, 40 (7), pp.25–39, pubmed.ncbi.nlm.nih.gov/30306398

4 Torelli and Manzoni (2005), 'Behavior during cluster headache'

5 NICE (2017), 'Headache – cluster', cks.nice.org.uk/topics/headache-cluster

6 ICHD-3 (2018), 'Headache or facial pain attributed to disorder of the cranium, neck, eyes, ears, nose, sinuses, teeth, mouth or other facial or cervical structure', ichd-3.org/11-headache-or-facial-pain-attributed-to-disorder-of-the-cranium-neck-eyes-ears-nose-sinuses-teeth-mouth-or-other-facial-or-cervical-structure/11-2-headache-attributed-to-disorder-of-the-neck/11-2-1-cervicogenic-headache

7 CSF Leak Association (n.d.), 'What is a CSF leak?', www.csfleak.info/what-is-a-cerebrospinal-fluid-csf-leak

8 Ehlers-Danlos Society (n.d.), 'What are the Ehlers-Danlos syndromes?', www.ehlers-danlos.com/what-is-eds

9 IIH UK (n.d.), 'What is IIH?', www.iih.org.uk/what-is-iih; National Eye Institute US (n.d.), 'Idiopathic intracranial hypertension', www.nei.nih.gov/learn-about-eye-health/eye-conditions-and-diseases/idiopathic-intracranial-hypertension

10 Anne Ducros and Marie-Germaine Bousser (2013), 'Thunderclap headache', *BMJ*, 346, art.e8557, www.bmj.com/content/346/bmj.e8557

11 P. A. McKinney (2004), 'Brain tumours: Incidence, survival, and aetiology', *Journal of Neurology, Neurosurgery & Psychiatry*, 75 (Suppl.2), pp.ii12–ii17, jnnp.bmj.com/content/75/suppl_2/ii12

12 ICHD-3 (2018), 'Visual snow', ichd-3.org/appendix/a1-migraine/a1-4-complications-of-migraine/a1-4-6-visual-snow

13 National Organization for Rare Disorders (n.d.), 'Visual snow syndrome', rarediseases.org/rare-diseases/visual-snow-syndrome

14. Managing Your Migraine

1 Richard B. Lipton, Daniel Serrano, Starr Holland et al. (2013), 'Barriers to the diagnosis and treatment of migraine: Effects of sex, income, and headache features', *Headache*, 53 (1), pp.81–92, pubmed.ncbi.nlm.nih.gov/23078241

2 David W. Dodick, Elizabeth W. Loder, Aubrey Manack Adams et al. (2016), 'Assessing barriers to chronic migraine consultation, diagnosis, and treatment: Results from the Chronic Migraine Epidemiology and Outcomes (CaMEO) Study', *Headache*, 56 (5), pp.821–34, www.ncbi.nlm.nih.gov/pmc/articles/PMC5084794

3 L. Kelman (2006), 'The broad treatment expectations of migraine patients', *Journal of Headache and Pain*, 7, pp.403–6, www.ncbi.nlm.nih.gov/pmc/articles/PMC3452218

4 Antonia F. H. Smelt, Mark A. Louter, Dennis A. Kies et al. (2014), 'What do patients consider to be the most important outcomes for effectiveness studies on migraine treatment? Results of a Delphi study', *PLoS One*, 9 (6), art.e98933, doi.org/10.1371/journal.pone.0098933

5 Richard B. Lipton and Walter F. Stewart (1999), 'Acute migraine therapy: Do doctors understand what patients with migraine want from therapy?', *Headache*, 39 (Suppl.2), pp.S20–6, headachejournal.onlinelibrary.wiley.com/doi/abs/10.1111/j.1526-4610.1999.00006.x

Further Reading and Resources

Information about treatments and guidelines

National Migraine Centre, www.nationalmigrainecentre.org.uk. UK charity offering appointments with specialist headache doctors. Factsheets are available on the website. Appointments with specialist headache doctors can be booked via a remote link. You can refer yourself. We also produce the *Heads Up* podcast on all things related to migraine and headache. Find out more at www.nationalmigrainecentre.org.uk/migraine-and-headaches/heads-up-podcast

British Association for the Study of Headache (BASH), www.bash.org.uk and www.headache.org.uk. Management guidelines for the treatment of headache disorders

International Headache Society (IHS), ihs-headache.org. The leading international organization for professionals interested in headache

NICE (National Institute for Health and Care Excellence), www.nice.org.uk. UK organization providing national guidelines for medical treatments, including migraine and cluster headache

SIGN (Scottish Intercollegiate Guidelines Network), www.sign.ac.uk. Scottish organization providing guidelines for medical treatments, including migraine

Patient advocacy organizations

In addition to the National Migraine Centre in the UK, the following work on behalf of people with migraine:

Migraine Trust, www.migrainetrust.org. A charity providing information and support to people with migraine in the UK

Migraine Again, www.migraineagain.com. Online support community

Migraine Australia, www.migraineaustralia.org

Migraine Canada, migrainecanada.org

Migraine Ireland, migraine.ie

European Migraine and Headache Alliance (EMHA), www.emhalliance.org

American Headache Society, americanheadachesociety.org

American Migraine Foundation, americanmigrainefoundation.org

Coalition for Headache and Migraine Patients (US), headachemigraine.org

Migraine diaries

National Migraine Centre, www.nationalmigrainecentre.org.uk/migraine-and-headaches/migraine-and-headache-diary. Downloadable monthly and annual diaries

Migraine Buddy, migrainebuddy.com

Migraine Trust, www.migrainetrust.org/living-with-migraine/coping-managing/keeping-a-migraine-diary

N1-headache, n1-headache.com

Learning about perceptions of migraine and stigma

Katherine Foxhall (2019), *Migraine: A History* (Baltimore: Johns Hopkins University Press)

Oliver Sacks (2012), *Migraine* (London: Picador)

Diet, nutrition and supplements

Felice Jacka (2019), *Brain Changer: How Diet Can Save Your Mental Health* (London: Yellow Kite)

British Dietetic Association glycaemic index (GI), www.bda.uk.com/resource/glycaemic-index.html

Exercise and posture

UK Chief Medical Officer, assets.publishing.service.gov.uk/government/uploads/system/uploads/attachment_data/file/829884/3-physical-activity-for-adults-and-older-adults.pdf. Physical-activity guidelines for people in the UK

US Department of Health and Human Services, health.gov/sites/default/files/2019–09/Physical_Activity_Guidelines_2nd_edition.pdf. American physical-activity guidelines

British Wheel of Yoga, www.bwy.org.uk

Pilates Foundation, www.pilatesfoundation.com

Tai Chi Union for Great Britain, www.taichiunion.com

Sleep

Kirstie Anderson (2018), *How to Beat Insomnia and Sleep Problems One Step at a Time: Using Evidence-based Low-intensity CBT* (London: Robinson)

Colin A. Espie (2006), *Overcoming Insomnia and Sleep Problems: A Self-Help Guide Using Cognitive Behavioral Techniques* (London: Robinson)

British Snoring Association, britishsnoring.co.uk

STOP-Bang, www.stopbang.ca/osa/screening.php. Questionnaire for help in diagnosing sleep apnoea

Mental-health and stress management for adults

Jon Kabat-Zinn (2013), *Full Catastrophe Living: How to Cope with Stress, Pain and Illness Using Mindfulness Meditation*, rev. edn (London: Piatkus)

Robert Lewin and Mike Bryson (2010), *Chronic Pain: The Pain Management Plan* (Melbourne, Yorks.: Npowered), www.pain-management-plan.co.uk

Pete Moore, The Pain Toolkit, www.paintoolkit.org

Kristin Neff (2011), *Self Compassion: Stop Beating Yourself Up and Leave Insecurity Behind* (London: Yellow Kite)

Mark Williams and Danny Penman (2011), *Mindfulness: A Practical Guide to Finding Peace in a Frantic World* (London: Piatkus). Includes CD with guided meditations

These apps and websites may have some useful free resources:

Mind UK, www.mind.org.uk

Calm, www.calm.com

Headspace, www.headspace.com

Andrew Johnson Meditation, www.andrewjohnson.co.uk

Black Dog Institute (Australia), www.blackdoginstitute.org.au

Smiling Mind (Australia), www.smilingmind.com.au

Stress and mental health for children and young people

Aaron Balick and Clotilde Szymanski (2020), *Keep Your Cool: How to Deal with Life's Worries and Stress* (London: Franklin Watts)

Dawn Heubner (2017), *Outsmarting Worry: An Older Kid's Guide to Managing Anxiety* (London: Jessica Kingsley). For children aged nine to thirteen

Suzy Reading (2019), *Stand Tall Like a Mountain: Mindfulness and Self-Care for Anxious Children and Worried Parents* (London: Aster)

Eline Snel (2019), *Sitting Still Like a Frog: Activity Book* (Boulder, CO: Shambhala). For children aged four to eight

Teen Breathe magazine, www.teenbreathe.co.uk

Relax Kids, www.relaxkids.com. Relaxation training for children and young people. Online video 'discovery calls' allow children to explore techniques

Young Minds, youngminds.org.uk. Charity supporting children and young people's mental health

These apps and websites may have some useful free resources:

Headspace for Kids, www.headspace.com/meditation/kids

Smiling Mind (Australia), www.smilingmind.com.au

Alternative therapies

British Acupuncture Council, www.acupuncture.org.uk

British Medical Acupuncture Society, www.medical-acupuncture.co.uk

British Society of Clinical Hypnosis, www.bsch.org.uk

American Society of Clinical Hypnosis, www.asch.net

General Osteopathic Council, www.osteopathy.org.uk/home

American Osteopathic Association, osteopathic.org

Pregnancy and breastfeeding

Breastfeeding Network (UK), www.breastfeedingnetwork.org.uk/migraines

bumps (Best Use of Medicines in Pregnancy), www.medicinesinpregnancy.org/ Medicine--pregnancy

LactMed (Drugs and Lactation Database), www.ncbi.nlm.nih.gov/books/ NBK501922/?report=classic

The menopause

Louise Newson (2021), *Preparing for the Perimenopause and Menopause,* Penguin Life Experts (London: Penguin)

British Menopause Society, thebms.org.uk. Includes factsheets on migraine and HRT, thebms.org.uk/publications/tools-for-clinicians/migraine-and-hrt

Australasian Menopause Society, www.menopause.org.au

North American Menopause Society, www.menopause.org

Work and benefits

Citizens Advice, www.citizensadvice.org.uk

Disability Rights UK, www.disabilityrightsuk.org

Migraine Trust employment advocacy service, www.migrainetrust.org/ wp-content/uploads/2015/09/employment-advocacy-toolkit-the-migraine-trust.pdf; phone 020 7631 6973

Turn2us, www.turn2us.org.uk. Benefits information and support

Education and schooling

National Migraine Centre, www.nationalmigrainecentre.org.uk/migraine-and-headaches/migraine-and-headache-factsheets/migraine-advice-to-schools. Leaflets to give to schools to explain migraine in your child

Department for Education, assets.publishing.service.gov.uk/government/uploads/system/uploads/attachment_data/file/349437/Supporting_pupils_with_medical_conditions_-_templates.docx. Guidelines around supporting children at school with medical conditions, including templates for communicating with schools

Migraine Trust, www.migrainetrust.org/living-with-migraine/asking-for-support/help-in-school. Leaflets to give to schools to explain migraine in your child

Royal College of GPs, School Policy Guidelines for School Students with Migraine and Troublesome Headache, www.gosh.nhs.uk/file/15301/download?token=4VwIcjZv. Leaflets to give to schools to explain migraine in your child

Seattle Children's Hospital, providernews.seattlechildrens.org/wp-content/uploads/PE2828.pdf. Some paediatric neurology departments produce sample letters with suggested accommodations that schools might make, this one being a good model

Managing migraine variants

Shin C. Beh (2020), *Victory over Vestibular Migraine: The ACTION Plan for Healing and Getting Your Life Back* (n.p.: independently published)

Organizations for people with other headache conditions

CSF Leak Association, www.csfleak.info

Ehlers-Danlos Society, www.ehlers-danlos.org

Hypermobility Syndromes Association (HMSA), www.hypermobility.org

IIH (Idiopathic Intracranial Hypertension) UK, www.iih.org.uk

OUCH (UK) (Organization for the Understanding of Cluster Headache), ouchuk.org

Support for people with brain tumours: Brains Trust, brainstrust.org.uk, and Brain Tumour Support, www.braintumoursupport.co.uk

Acknowledgements

I would very much like to thank Robin Dennis, Lydia Yadi and Susannah Bennett and the team at Penguin Random House for the opportunity and their encouragement and guidance in writing this book.

Thanks to my colleagues Dr Jessica Briscoe, Dr Nazeli Manyukan, Dr Carole Tallon, Prof. Paul Booton, Dr Richard Wood, Dr Sarah Miller, Swati Raina and Charlotte Burr O'Kane for all their amazing work and to all in the dedicated team at the National Migraine Centre. Thanks to all the wonderful guests who have shared their stories and expertise on our *Heads Up* podcast too.

Many thanks too for great support for me and people with migraine from Dr Kate Barnes, Dr Louise Rusk, Dr David Kernick, Dr David Watson, Dr Mark Weatherall and Professor Anne Macgregor.

Thanks always to these wonderful people: Bernard, Tom, Liz, Allie, Jess Bleackley, Sue Hope, Isabelle McKenna, Sue Rhodes and Sarah Armitage.

And finally I would like to say a huge thank you to all the patients from whom I have learned, and continue to learn, so much over the years.